Diagnosing and Managing Temporomandibular Joint Conditions

Edited by Vladimír Machoň

Published in London, United Kingdom

Diagnosing and Managing Temporomandibular Joint Conditions
http://dx.doi.org/10.5772/intechopen.1001690
Edited by Vladimír Machoň

Contributors
Aly Mohamed Atteya, Annalisa Pollice, Arturo Ivan Espinosa Carlos, Carmelo Consiglio, Ciro Emiliano Boschetti, Daniela Chroustová, Davide Morlando, David Guida, David J. Psutka, Fabrizio Chirico, Gianpaolo Tartaro, Giuseppe Colella, Gunjan Pani, Ivo Ferrieri, Leandro Díez-Suárez, Luigi Rugge, Mario Santagata, Michal Beňo, Neha Nainoor, Roberta Magliulo, Roberta Sivo, Rodrigo Garay Symor, Ryan J. McCoy, Salvatore D'Amato, Vladimír Machoň

First published in London, United Kingdom, 2025 by IntechOpen
IntechOpen is the global imprint of INTECHOPEN LIMITED, registered in England and Wales, registration number: 11086078, 167-169 Great Portland Street, London, W1W 5PF, United Kingdom

For EU product safety concerns: IN TECH d.o.o., Prolaz Marije Krucifikse Kozulić 3, 51000 Rijeka, Croatia, info@intechopen.com or visit our website at intechopen.com.

British Library Cataloguing-in-Publication Data
A catalogue record for this book is available from the British Library

Diagnosing and Managing Temporomandibular Joint Conditions
Edited by Vladimír Machoň
p. cm.
Print ISBN 978-0-85466-662-1
Online ISBN 978-0-85466-661-4
eBook (PDF) ISBN 978-0-85466-663-8

If disposing of this product, please recycle the paper responsibly.

Meet the editor

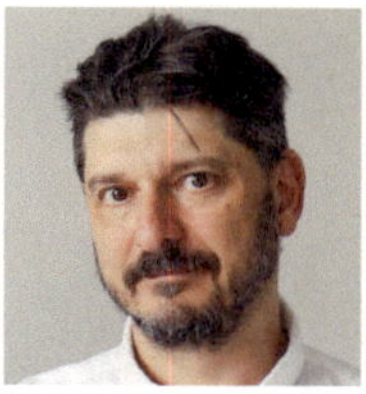

Dr. Vladimír Machoň was born in 1973 in Pilsen. He is a graduate of Masaryk University in Brno, Czech Republic, where he earned degrees in both dentistry and general medicine. Dr. Machoň has established himself as a leading TMJ (temporomandibular joint) surgeon and is actively involved in publishing and lecturing on managing TMJ disorders. He is a founding member of the European Society of TMJ Surgeons (ESTMJS).

Contents

Preface

The temporomandibular joint (TMJ) is one of the most stressed joints in the human body. It is a paired joint (two joints connected by the lower jaw) and a compound joint (there is a disc between the head and the socket). The temporomandibular joint disease affects 15–20% of the population, according to some studies, up to 30%. It is, therefore, a common disease.

As time evolves, so does the view of temporomandibular joint disease, its etiology and management. The view that associated temporomandibular joint disease with occlusal disorders alone has long been abandoned. Today's view is a whole-body view; the joint is seen as part of the whole body. Similar pathological factors apply to it as to other joints. Similar rules of therapy apply to it, as in orthopaedics. Thus, it is unsurprising that lavage, arthroscopy, and total joint replacements are performed for some TMJ disorders.

This book aims to contribute to current knowledge in diagnosing and managing TMJ disease. Individual chapters cover imaging techniques, myofascial pain, minimally invasive techniques, and operative arthroscopy. The book includes two chapters on condylar head changes regarding condylar resorption and condylar hyperplasia. The book concludes with the issues of TMJ reconstruction with total joint replacement.

This book is intended for dentists, oral surgeons, maxillofacial surgeons, ENT physicians, students, and anyone interested in TMJ disease.

My thanks go to all the authors of each chapter. And I also thank Antonija Grgeč (IntechOpen Publishing Process Manager) for her help in completing this book.

Vladimir Machoň
TMJ Surgeon,
Department Oral Maxillofacial Surgery,
Charles University and Faculty Hospital Prague,
Prague, Czech Republic

Department of Oral Maxillofacial Surgery,
Hospital České Budějovice,
České Budějovice, Czech Republic

Chapter 1

Imaging of Temporomandibular Joint

Neha Nainoor and Gunjan Pani

Abstract

The temporomandibular joint (TMJ) is crucial for proper mouth function, and issues with it can cause significant discomfort and reduce the quality of life for those affected. Over the years, TMJ imaging has advanced to enhance overall patient care, treatment planning, and diagnostic accuracy. Temporomandibular joint disorders (TMD) are complex and poorly understood conditions characterized by pain in the affected area and restricted jaw movements. Radiographic examination is a key part of the standard clinical assessment for patients with TMDs. Conventional imaging methods like CT scans and X-rays are being replaced by advanced techniques such as MRI, which provides superior visualization of soft tissues and higher diagnostic accuracy, especially with contrast-enhanced high-resolution MRI. The integration of three-dimensional (3D) imaging techniques, such as multi-detector CT (MDCT) and cone-beam computed tomography (CBCT), has reshaped the assessment of TMJ anatomy and pathology. This combination enables the visualization of the joint in multiple thin sections, aiding in identifying minor structural abnormalities. Additionally, techniques like ultrasound (USG) provide real-time insights into dynamic TMJ function, offering valuable information on joint movement and biomechanics. Despite these significant advancements, challenges persist, including the need for standardized imaging protocols, access to advanced technologies, and ongoing research to validate the clinical usefulness of newer imaging methods.

Keywords: TMJ imaging, temporomandibular joint, radiographic investigation, TMJ disorders, CT, CBCT, MRI, USG

1. Introduction

The temporomandibular joint (TMJ) serves as a critical component of the craniofacial complex, facilitating essential functions such as mastication, speech, and facial expression. Pathological conditions affecting the TMJ, collectively known as temporomandibular joint disorders (TMD), can lead to debilitating pain, restricted jaw movement, and a decline in overall quality of life. Accurate diagnosis and effective management of TMJ disorders necessitate advanced imaging techniques that can provide detailed anatomical and functional information.

Temporomandibular joint (TMJ) pain is prevalent in the general population, with only 3–7% of patients seeking medical attention [1, 2].

TMDs often involve structural and functional changes in the TMJ and adjacent structures like muscles of mastication, ligaments, teeth, and periodontal tissue [3].

In recent years, there has been a remarkable surge in technological advancements within the field of medical imaging, offering clinicians clear insights into the intricacies of the TMJ. These developments have not only enhanced the ability to visualize the joint's structures but also revolutionized our understanding of dynamic functional aspects. Different imaging modalities are available to image the TMJ, each with inherent strengths and weaknesses [4].

Traditional imaging methods, such as plain radiography and computed tomography (CT), have long been employed for TMD cases. While these techniques have proven valuable, the advent of magnetic resonance imaging (MRI) has brought an evolution to this field. MRI's ability to provide high-resolution, multi-planar, thin-sectioned images without ionizing radiation makes it particularly well-suited for capturing the intricate soft tissue anatomy of the TMJ, including the articular disc, ligaments, and surrounding musculature [5].

Beyond conventional imaging, three-dimensional (3D) technologies, such as cone-beam computed tomography (CBCT) and multi-detector CT (MDCT) have opened in a new era of precision in TMJ evaluation. These modalities offer the slightest detail into bony anatomy, allowing clinicians to identify subtle structural abnormalities and facilitating the development of customized treatment strategies. Moreover, advanced contrast-enhanced MRI techniques contribute to even superior diagnostic accuracy by highlighting specific pathological features [6, 7].

Ultrasound and functional imaging methods, have added a dynamic dimension to TMJ assessment. Real-time visualization of joint movements and biomechanics provides clinicians with invaluable information for a comprehensive understanding of TMJ function. This real-time data can aid in the diagnosis of conditions related to joint dynamics, leading to more effective and targeted interventions [8].

While these advancements hold immense promise, challenges do persist, including the standardization of imaging protocols, accessibility to cutting-edge technologies for developing nations and the need for continued research to validate the clinical efficacy of these newer imaging modalities. This exploration of recent advancements in TMJ imaging sets the stage for a more in-depth examination of each modality's strengths and weaknesses and the potential contributions to advancing the field of maxillofacial diagnostics and therapeutics.

2. Temporomandibular radiography

The use of conventional radiography for the accurate evaluation of the TMJ is restricted by the presence of structure superimposition. There are various views that demonstrate the temporomandibular joint. Structure superimposition limits the use of conventional radiography for proper TMJ examination. There are various views that demonstrate the temporomandibular joint.

- Trans-Cranial View

- Trans-pharyngeal View

- Trans-orbital View
- Reverse Towne's Projection

2.1 Trans-cranial view

It is also known as Lindblom's view. This technique is particularly effective in detecting arthritic changes on the articular surface, assessing the bony relationship of the joint, despite not detecting changes on the central and medial surfaces [9–11]. This view is taken with the patient's mouth in three positions (**Figures 1** and **2**).

1. Open mouth.
2. Rest position.
3. Closed mouth.

2.1.1 Indications

1. To study the position of the condyles in the glenoid fossa.

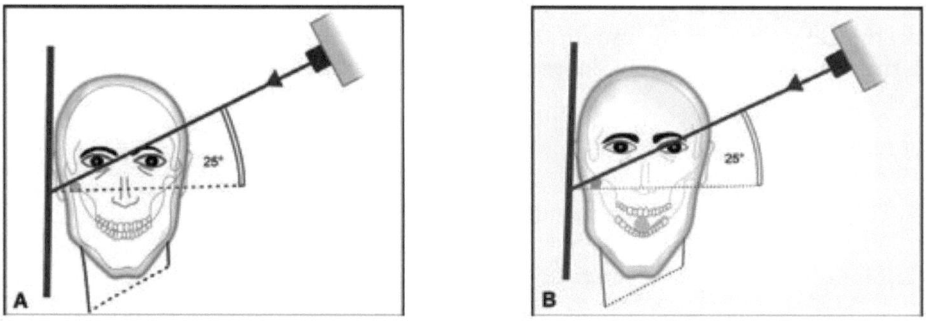

Figure 1.
Transcranial projection, the central ray is oriented at a 25° positive angle and 20° anteriorly centered over the TMJ of interest, (A) Mouth closed. (B) Mouth open.

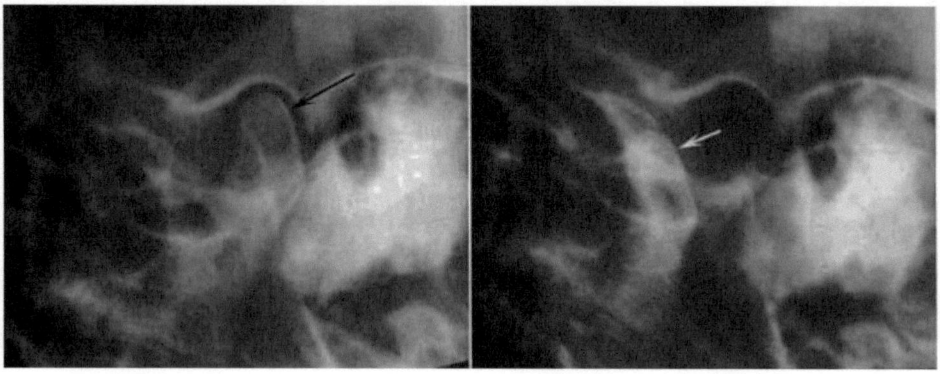

Figure 2.
Transcranial view – Mouth closed position transcranial view – Mouth open position.

2. To study the joint space, i.e. the space between the articulating surfaces of the glenoid fossa and the condyles for either partial or complete obliteration (ankylosis).

3. To study antero-posterior mobility. (Hypermobility, i.e. dislocation and subluxation.)

4. To study osseous change such as flattening in arthritis.

2.1.2 Limitations

- Sub-condylar fractures cannot be seen because of superimposition of ipsilateral petrous bone and posterior clinoid process of sella turcica on the neck of the condyle.

- The radiograph shows only the lateral part of the joint space.

2.2 Trans-pharyngeal view

It is also known as Infracranial or McQueen Dell Technique (**Figures 3** and **4**).

The view is a lateral projection of the medial surface of the condylar head and neck, typically taken in the mouth open position, allowing the joint to be projected into the nasopharynx shadow, increasing joint contrast [9–11].

2.2.1 Indications

1. TMJ pain dysfunction syndrome

2. Joint disease such as osteoarthritis and rheumatoid arthritis.

3. Pathological conditions affecting the condylar head such as cysts or tumors.

4. Condylar head and neck fractures [10].

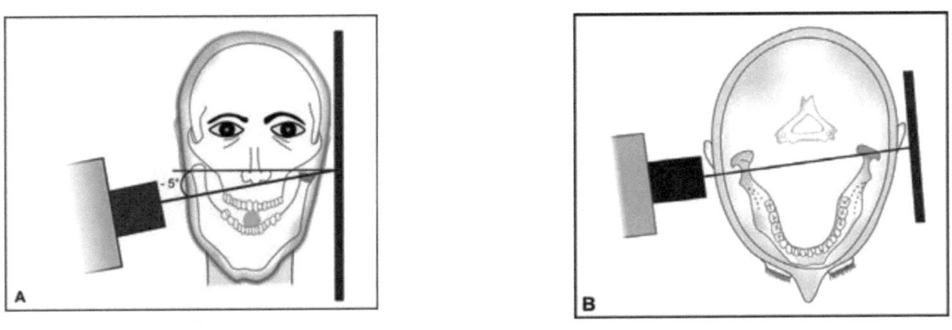

Figure 3.
(A) Trans-pharyngeal projection. The central ray is oriented superiorly 5° to 10° and posteriorly approximately 10°, centered over the TMJ of interest. The mandible is positioned at maximal opening. (B) Trans-pharyngeal projection showing positioning from above, showing the X-ray beam aimed slightly posteriorly across the pharynx.

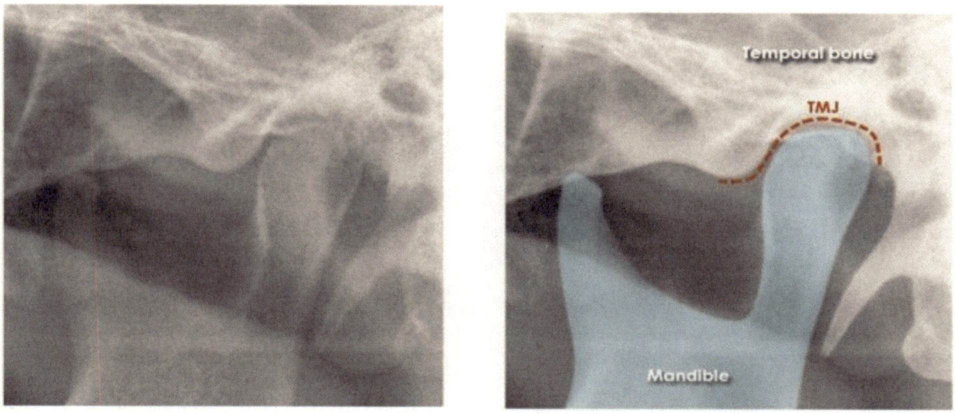

Figure 4.
Trans-pharyngeal view.

2.3 Trans-orbital view (Zimmer projection)

This is the conventional frontal TM joint projection is highly effective in delineating joints with minimal super impositions, resulting in a relatively true 'enface' projection (**Figure 5**).

2.3.1 Indications

1. To study medio-lateral displacement of the condyle.
2. To study superior surfaces of the condyle for osteophytes, etc.
3. To study the relationship of the condyle to the articular eminence in the mediolateral plane.[5]

2.4 Reverse Towne's

This projection is useful in viewing the condylar head and neck. The original Towne's view, an AP projection, was intended to show the occipital region and

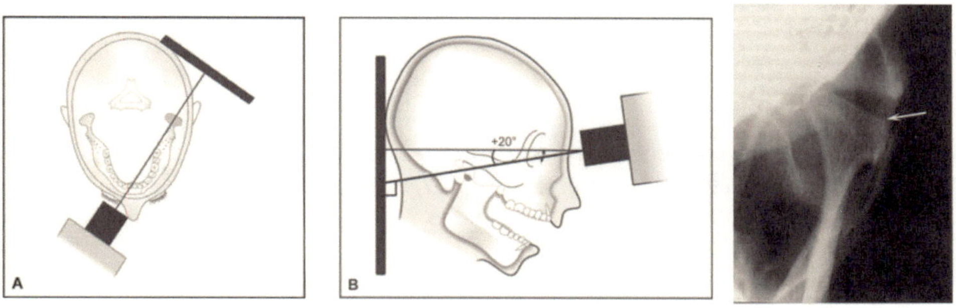

Figure 5.
Trans-orbital projection. The central ray is oriented downward approximately 20° and laterally approximately 30° through the contralateral orbit, centered over the TMJ of interest.

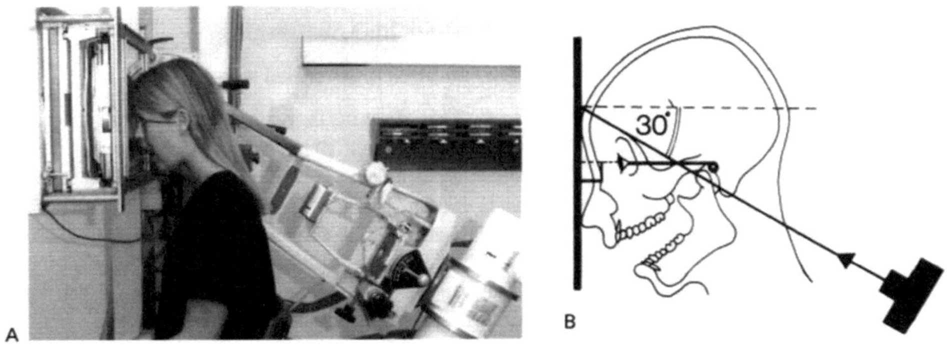

Figure 6.
(A) The patient is in a forehead-nose position with an open mouth and an X-ray beam aimed upwards at 30°, as shown in the reverse Towne's projection positioning diagram; (B) the radiographic baseline is horizontal and perpendicular to the film.

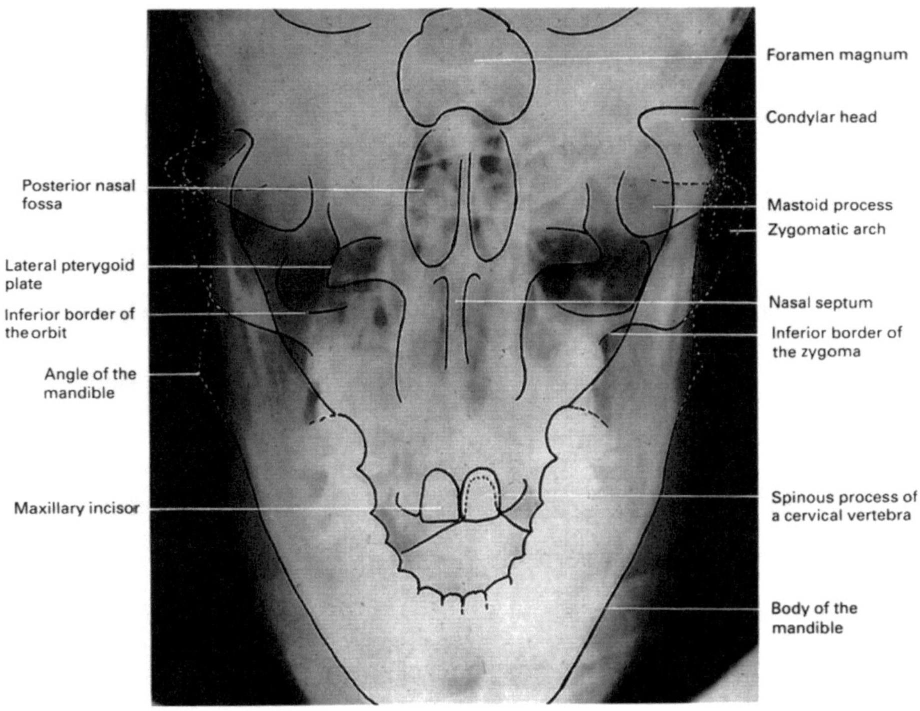

Figure 7.
Reverse Towne's view.

condyles, but due to conventional dental skull views being taken in the PA direction, the reverse Towne's (PA) projection is used (**Figures 6** and 7) [11].

2.4.1 Indications

- High condylar necks fractures
- Intra-capsular TMJ fractures

- Examining the quality of condylar head articular surfaces in TMJ disorders

- Condylar hypoplasia or hyperplasia.

3. Computed tomography (CT)

For the assessment of the TMJ, computed tomography (CT) has shown to be an invaluable tool. CT has been employed in the detection of uncommon disorders such synovial osteochondromatosis as well as bony abnormalities of the TMJ. A wide range of osseous pathological alterations, including osteophytes, condylar erosion, fractures, ankylosis, dislocation, internal disc derangement diagnosis, and growth anomalies such condylar hyperplasia, can be well visualized with CT.

Research conducted on autopsy specimens revealed that CT has a 100% specificity, 100% positive predictive value, and 78% negative predictive value for identifying alterations in the bone [12]. Nevertheless, the very high radiation dose, equipment accessibility, and expensive cost have restricted it's widespread use in TMJ evaluation [11, 13].

Multi-detector CT (MDCT) is more widely available and better tolerated. In both closed and open mouth postures, MDCT is carried out without the need for intravenous or intra-articular contrast media. Multi-planar reconstructions are performed

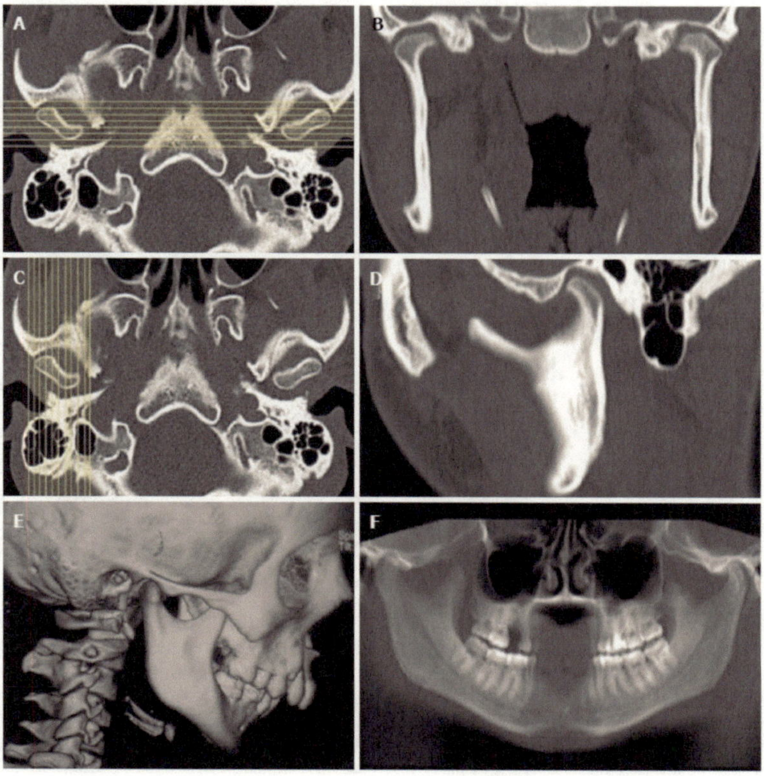

Figure 8.
Technique of reconstruction. A, B: Sagittal images are reconstructed perpendicular to the glenoid fossa plane.; C, D: Reconstructed coronal pictures are oriented perpendicularly to the sagittal image plane.; E, F: The 3D reformatted and reassembled panoramic image accurately depicts the anatomy of the joint. (Source: [15].)

using bone and soft-tissue techniques in the coronal oblique, parallel to the long axis of the mandibular condyle and sagittal oblique planes, perpendicular to the long axis of the mandibular condyle [14].

For acquisition, the slice thickness and interval should be between 0.5 and 1 mm. Coronal images are reconstructed parallel to the mandibular condyles, with a slice thickness and inter-slice gap of 2–3 mm. Sagittal images are reconstructed from the raw data perpendicular to the plane of mandibular condyles as seen on axial plane (**Figure 8**) [15].

The multi-planar reconstructions are examined using a DICOM viewer (**Figure 8**). In order to identify any anomalies in the imaging volume, that might be incidental or the cause of symptoms resembling TMJ dysfunction, the source axial images are also examined. It has been discovered that MDCT is a helpful imaging test for the accurate diagnosis of internal disc derangement, arthritis, and other various TMJ disorders [14]. The normal appearance of the TMJ on a CT scan is as shown in **Figure 9**.

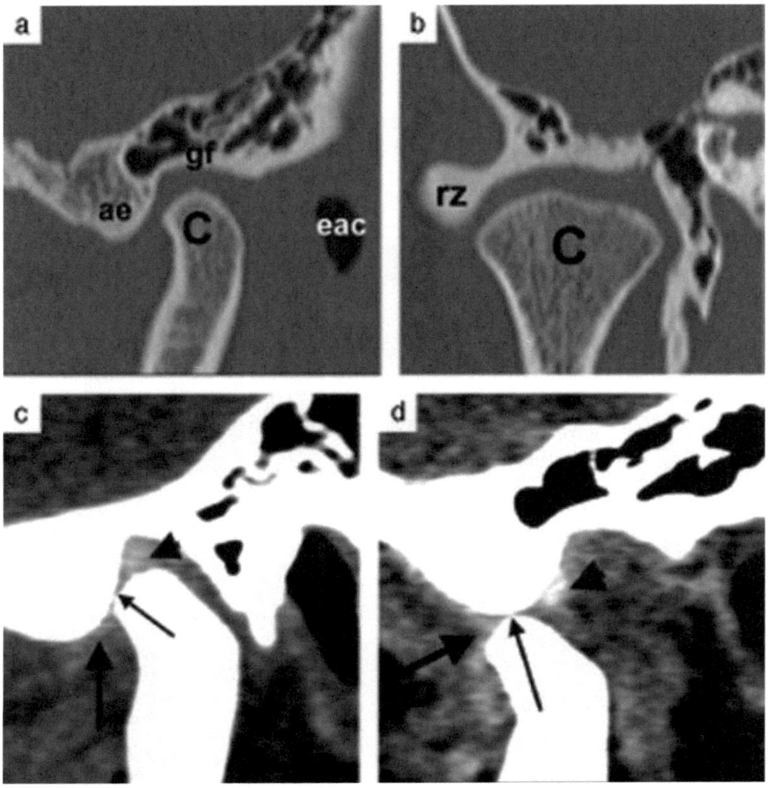

Figure 9.
Normal CT anatomy of the temporomandibular joint. (a) The mandibular condyle (C) is seated inside the glenoid fossa (gf) of the temporal bone in this oblique sagittal reconstruction at the bone window, created with the use of a bone reconstruction algorithm. The external auditory canal (eac) is posterior to the temporal bone's articular eminence (ae). (b) A bone reconstruction algorithm is used for oblique coronal reconstruction at the bone window. The coronal dimension of the condyle is broad. The zygomatic process's base is located laterally (rz). (c) Oblique sagittal reconstruction in the closed-mouth position employing soft-tissue windows and a soft-tissue reconstruction method. The anterior band (thick arrow) and posterior band (arrowhead) are easily apparent. The thin intermediate zone (thin arrow) is located at the narrowest point between the condyle and the articular eminence. The posterior boundary of the posterior band is often located at the 12 o'clock position. (d) Soft-tissue oblique sagittal reconstruction in an open mouth position. The condyle has moved anteriorly onto the articular eminence, causing the disc to shift anteriorly as well. The anterior band (thick arrow), posterior band (arrowhead), and intermediate zone (thin arrow) are again illustrated.

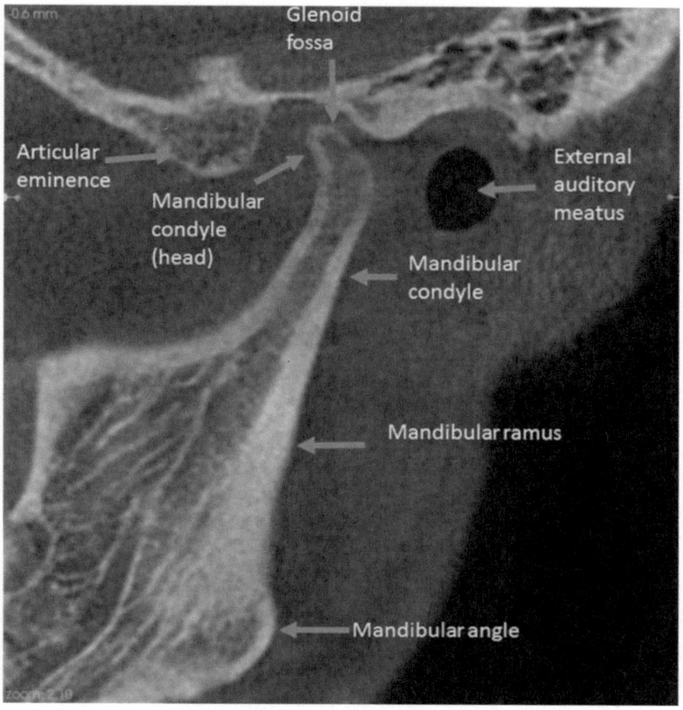

Figure 10.
Normal anatomy of TMJ as viewed on CBCT image. (Source: [19]).

4. Cone beam computed tomography (CBCT)

Cone beam CT (CBCT), introduced in 1982, is a low-dose technique for visualizing bony structures in the head and neck. Despite limitations like high radiation doses and long scanning times, CBCT offers high spatial resolution and less scanning time, making it the preferred imaging modality for maxilla-mandibular regions. Compared to multi-slice CT, CBCT produces high-resolution multi-planar images with a reduced dose of radiation [12]. CBCT has a higher sensitivity of 0.80 for detecting degenerative TMJ changes, with diagnostic accuracy dependent on defect size, with high sensitivity for condylar defects compared to CT [7, 16]. Caruso et al.'s study suggests that CBCT 3D Imaging improves detection of changes in condylar shape, and clarifies condyle position in the glenoid fossa [17].

Imaging diagnosis is crucial for evaluating TMJ conditions, assessing bone structures, and assessing the position of the condyle within the glenoid cavity. It helps confirm the progression of disorders and evaluate treatment effects. Other factors to consider include condylar fractures, neoplasms, malformations, and potential solutions to cranial vault continuity [18]. Normal anatomy of TMJ on a CBCT is as shown in **Figure 10**.

5. Magnetic resonance imaging (MRI)

MRI, developed in 1977, is a non-invasive imaging technique that uses low-frequency radio waves to produce images. It uses protons to change position, producing signals

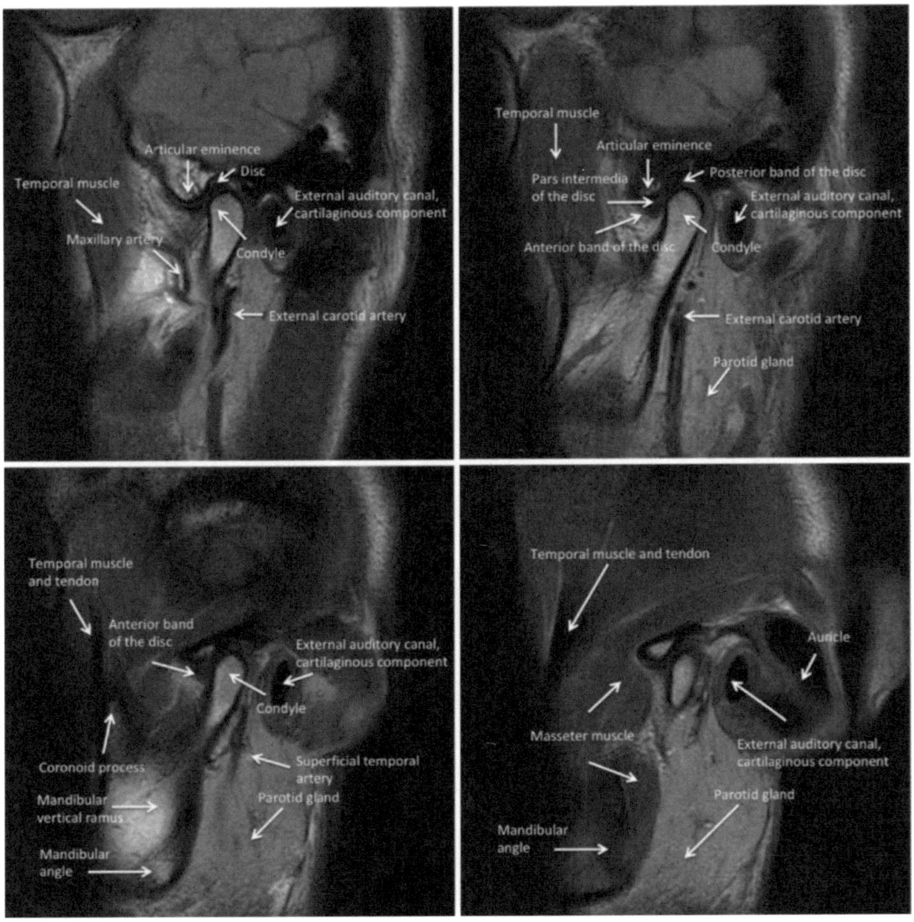

Figure 11.
Normal anatomy of TMJ on an MRI image.

based on tissue density. Tissue rich in water emits a hyper-signal, producing clear images, while tissues lacking water emit a hypo-signal, producing dark images. As a result, components richer in water, including muscle and fat, send intermediate signals that produce images in shades of gray, while cortical bone, which is poor in water, emits a hyposignal that results in a dark image [4]. MRI scans reveal high T1 signal intensity in condyle marrow fat, low signal intensity in cortical bone and disk due to low proton density and short T2, and high T2 and PD signal intensity in central disk (**Figure 11**) [8].

MRI of the TMJ captures the disk and its relation to the condylar head, indicating TMJ dysfunction. Diagnosis depends on factors like joint effusion, ruptured retro-discal layers, and thickening of lateral pterygoid muscle attachment. Advanced degenerative joint disease is characterized by osteoarthritic changes. MRI is used to identify disk injuries, joint effusion, and differentiate between synovial proliferation and joint effusion. Gadolinium-enhanced MRI distinguishes proliferating synovium from joint effusion [9].

6. TMJ arthrography

Arthrography of the TM joint examines soft tissue state, including disk integrity and position, and provides evidence of internal disk derangement or perforation.

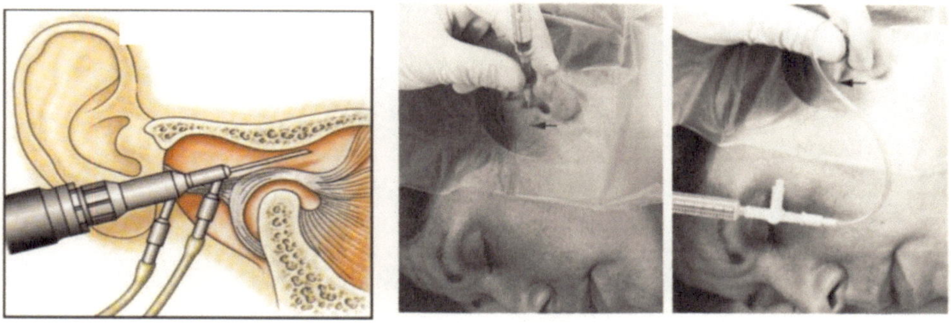

Figure 12.
Arthrographic technique. Left, the TMJ arthrogram site as well as the route for inserting the angiocatheter into the lower joint space are displayed. A sterile drape is placed over the preauricular area, and a 22-gauge angiocatheter is positioned perpendicular to the skin's surface (arrow at the puncture site). The operator pushes the tool into the tissue until it makes touch with the condyle's posterolateral surface. The angiocatheter would be positioned somewhat superior and anterior using the same approach, but with a reasonably broad opening. Right, the angiocatheter hub (arrow at the puncture site) is attached to the tube and syringe for the contrast medium injection. Slowly injecting contrast is done while being periodically observed via a fluoroscope. A stopcock at the synringe's tip seals the system when the contrast agent is injected.

It's useful for diagnosing cases with minimal bone damage and clinical evidence suggesting disk derangement [10].

Dr. Fleming Norgaard introduced positive contrast agent in 1947 for TMJ visualization, but it wasn't globally acclaimed until 1970 when Wilkes unmasked it in the US, by the inoculation of a radiopaque contrast material into the temporomandibular joint spaces, leading to single and double contrast techniques [20].

Procedure: TM joint arthrography involves catheterizing the upper and lower joint spaces and injecting 0.5–1 ml of radiographic contrast media, typically iodine compounds, into the lower and upper spaces (**Figure 12**) [10]. The contrast medium, containing 300 mg iodine/mL, should be administered in small amounts to the TMJ (1.5-2 ml), reducing the risk of idiosyncratic reactions as it is injected only into the joint compartments [21]. After joint space opacification, a series of radiographs/CBCT

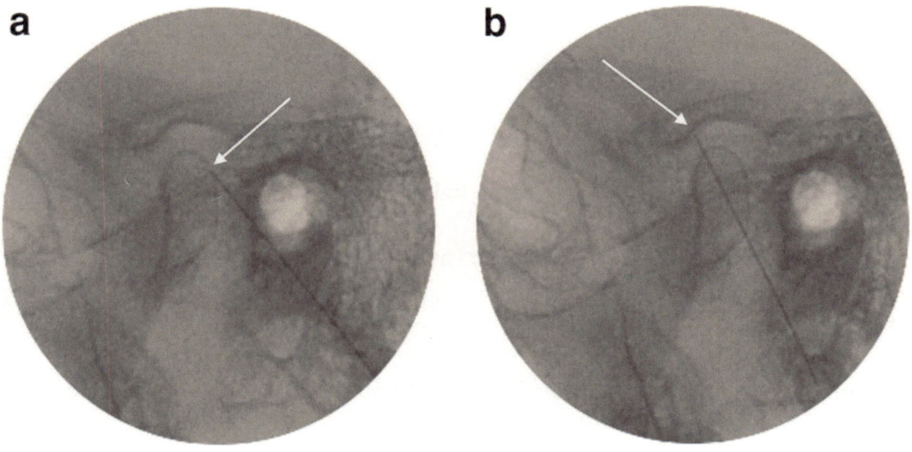

Figure 13.
(a) The placement of the needle during the anesthetic injection before the TMJ (left side) arthrography. Anesthesia is administered by placing the needle tip in close proximity to the upper posterior region of the lateral pole of the condyle. (b) A needle is positioned in close proximity to the articular tubercle's posterior surface to administer anesthetic before injecting contrast material into the upper joint compartment.

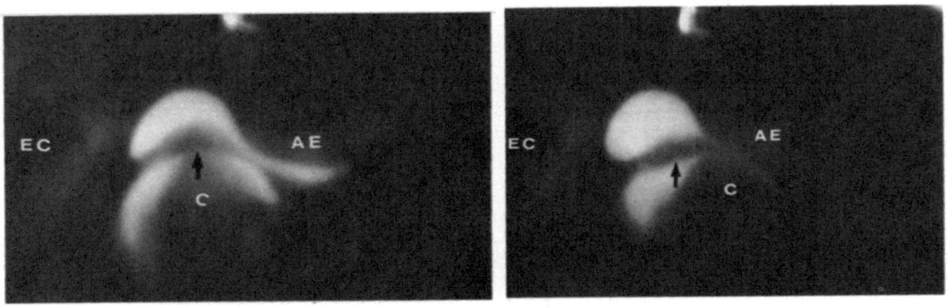

Figure 14.
Normal temporomandibular arthrogram. Left, both upper and lower joint spaces are moderately opacified; jaws are opened approximately one fingerbreadth of interincisal distance. Portion of contrast medium is seen in anterior recesses. Posterior band (arrow) of disk is positioned directly above condyle. Right, jaws are opened farther and condyle is anteriorly translated to greater extent, obliterating contrast in both anterior recesses. Posterior band of disk (arrow) trails behind condyle. C, condyle; AE, articular eminence; EC, external ear canal.

(**Figures 13** and **14**) are obtained with the jaws closed and in graduated stages of opening. Since there is not a known normal circumstance in which there is contact between the superior and inferior joint spaces, the disk appears as a radiolucent vacuum between two opaque regions of contrast media [10].

6.1 Indications

- Symptoms of TMJ arthralgia/arthritis include pain during jaw movement and restricted opening.
- Conservative treatments such non-steroid anti-inflammatory medications, occlusal splints, and jaw exercises that did not significantly reduce pain.
- Indications of internal derangement or adhesion [21].

6.2 Diagnostic information obtained

- Dynamic information on joint components and disk movement.
- Static images of components with closed and open mouths.
- Observation of anterior or anteromedial disk displacement (**Figure 15**).
- Examination of disk integrity, perforations presence.

6.3 Advantages

- Fluoroscopically, abnormalities like discontinuation, any tear or adhesion can be appreciated. Action of the articular disc and fluid accumulation can be seen as well.
- Simultaneous sampling of synovial fluid and joint lavage.
- Enhancement of disc shape and position through tomography.

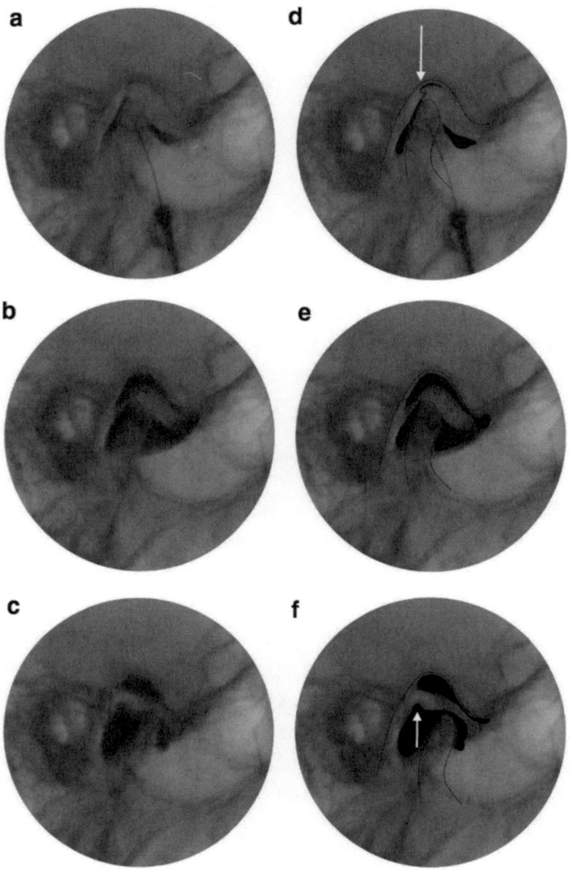

Figure 15.
TMJ arthrography (right side) demonstrates anterior disc displacement, reduction, and posterior attachment perforation. (a–c) an oblique transcranial projection that displays the joint's lateral aspect. (d–f) corresponding photos with the joint components indicated and contrast media emphasized. (a, d) when the mouth is closed, a rupture in the disc's posterior attachment allows contrast material to flow into the upper compartment (arrow). When the mouth is closed, both compartments loaded with contrast have an anterior disc displacement (b, e). (c, f) In the open mouth position, the disc is decreased and a posterior attachment defect is visible (arrow).

- Diagnosis of joint mice.
- Distinguishing internal derangement and inflammation.

6.4 Disadvantages

- Excludes severely deformed disc.
- Interpretation challenges due to medial or lateral articular disc displacements.
- Potential significant radiation exposure.
- Common procedure hitches: contrast medium extravasation, joint pain, minimal with non-ionic contrast media [20].

- Large needles and cannulas can be a cause of parotitis in arthrography.
- Transient facial paralysis is another complication when there is vigorous infiltration of lidocaine.

7. Ultrasonography (USG)

Ultrasonography (USG) is a cost-effective, non-invasive imaging method used for abdominal and extremity imaging. It was first used for diagnosing TMJ disorders in 1991, and with advancements in higher frequency probes and higher resolution devices, its scope is promising [22].

7.1 Ultrasound protocol

Conventional US transducer positions, in both closed-mouth (**Figure 16** A,C) and open-mouth (**Figure 16** B,D) positions, are parallel to the ramus of the mandible and the Frankfort horizontal plane, which is a plane that connects the highest point of the external auditory canal with the lowest point on the lower margin of the orbit. Normal transverse section ultrasound image of the mandible in the closed (E) and open (F) mouth positions.

The articular disk's normal ultrasound appearance in the sagittal plane is an inverted hypoechoic C-shaped structure, as seen by the red circle. During the mouth opening, the mandibular condyle moves anteriorly, as indicated by the distance between the center of the condylar oval at the two positions (yellow dotted line) (**Figure 16**). In normal anatomy, the disk appears centrally in relation to the center of the mandibular condyle, however in pathological findings, it may be moved anteriorly or posteriorly (**Figure 17**) [23]. US effusion diagnosis was found to be more accurate than the gold standard MRI.

Emshoff et al. [24] used a 7.5 MHz transducer, which demonstrated a sensitivity of 40–50% and specificity of 70%. Diagnostic accuracy was acceptable in both positions,

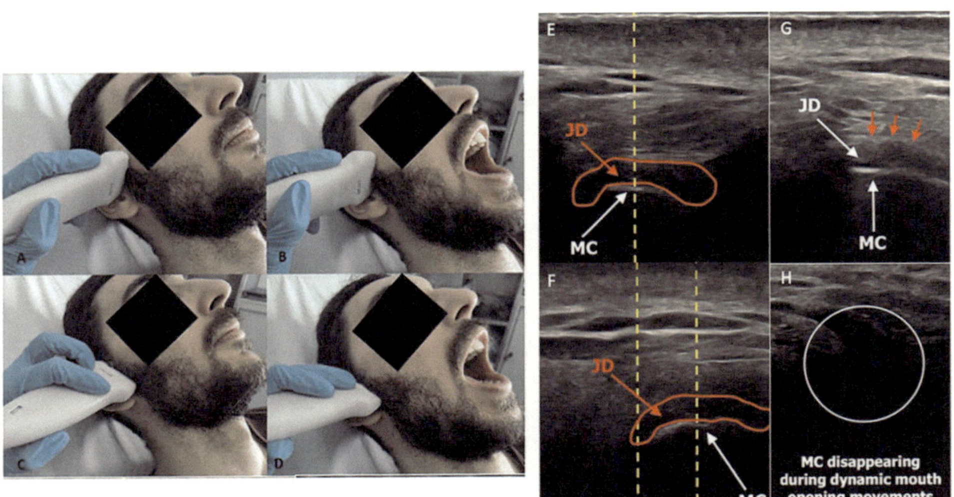

Figure 16.
The TMJ is seen in a normal ultrasound scan in both the open-mouth (H) and closed-mouth (G) positions. The articular capsule is indicated by red arrows. Joint disk (JD) and mandibular condyle (MC).

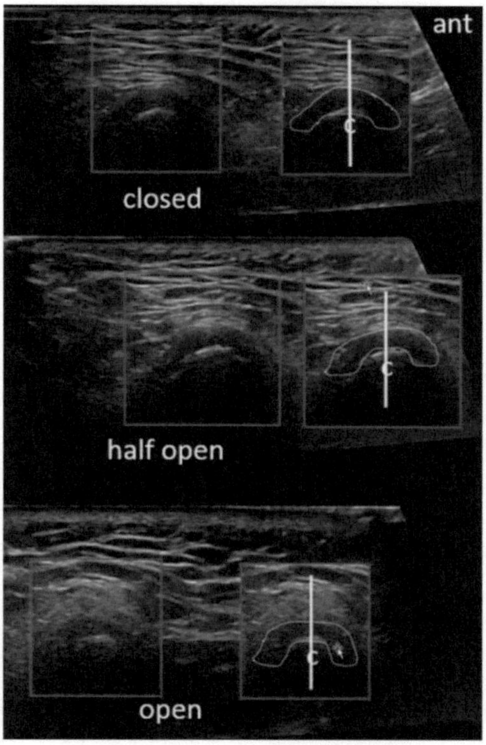

Figure 17.
On normal ultrasonography, the articular disc appears in the sagittal plane as an inverted hypoechoic c-shaped structure. Throughout the closed-mouth, half-open-mouth, and fully-open-mouth views, the disc maintains a consistent central appearance in relation to the center of the condyle, "c," which is delineated by a central vertical line. The articular disc's anterior ("ant") and posterior bands appear to be symmetrical in size when viewed from the center of the condyle. A focused annotated view was supplied to help visibility, with the articular disc highlighted with a dotted contour.

but sensitivity decreased from closed to open mouth. In contrast, specificity increased from closed to open mouth position. Progressive use of transducers with higher frequencies, of 10 MHz or more, results in improved sensitivity, ranging from 60–90% [23]. Jank et al. [25] discovered that HR-US may detect TMJ pathology even before clinical symptoms manifested, which is especially important in the younger population to prevent further damage.

7.2 Indications

Injuries and inflammation of the tendons, ligaments, soft tissues, and bones should be investigated using US, particularly in cases of post-traumatic pain syndromes, restricted joint mobility, and post-traumatic disorders. Moreover, the diagnosis of degenerative illnesses and interventional procedure cases (biopsies, punctures, and intra-articular injections) can be aided by ultrasound scanning.

7.3 Advantages

- Allows real-time motion observation.

- Helps localize imaging to patient-directed pain regions.
- Evaluates claustrophobic patients with non-MRI compatible stents and implants.
- Visualizes cortical osseous defects like osteophytes and erosions.
- Partial limitation by patient body habitus.
- Allows acoustic windows by adjacent osseous structures.

7.4 Disadvantages

- Difficulty in visualizing medial and lateral disc displacements.
- Inadequate visualization of perforations and adhesions.
- Inability to visualize subcortical osseous abnormalities.
- Inherent operator dependence and learning curve.

8. Nucleide imaging

Nucleide imaging uses radioactive isotopes to examine the entire maxillofacial region and TMJ, detecting active inflammatory processes [26]. This method is unique in assessing physiologic changes due to biochemical alteration. It relies on the radiotracer method, which assumes that radioactive atoms or molecules in an organism behave identically to their stable counterparts due to their chemical indistinguishability [27]. Depending on the registration methods, the nuclear imaging methods are of three types:

a. Scintigraphy

b. Single photon emission computed tomography (SPECT)

c. Positron Emission Tomography (PET)

8.1 Scintigraphy

Traditional radiographs and advanced imaging techniques have limitations in determining structural changes, but bone scintigraphy can aid in diagnosing TMJ disease activity, determining remodeling and inflammation, and managing the condition. Bone scintigraphy involves injecting technetium diphosphonate 99 mTC into the circulation, and metabolic images are obtained 2–3 hours post-injection. An intravenous dose of 99 mTC is determined by 740 MBq × body weight/70 kg [28].

The bone tracer complex, 99 mTC, is activated by blood flow and calcium-containing crystals binding to phosphate. It produces c-radiation, detected by a scintillation camera indicating bone metabolic activity. Positive scans correlate with clinical signs and symptoms (**Figure 18**). However, a bone scan is non-specific and may show conditions like growth, healing bone, infection, arthritic changes, or tumors [29].

Bone scintigraphy detects active joint changes, stability, and inflammation, which can influence treatment. Its ability to detect or rule out remodeling in the TMJ

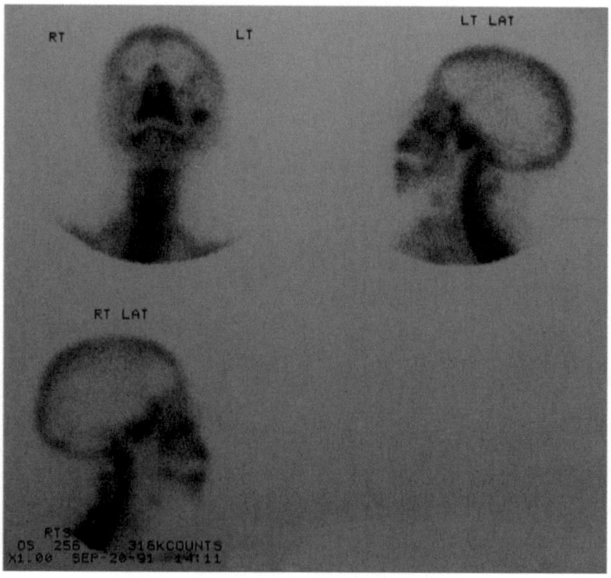

Figure 18.
Bone scintigraphy showing increased uptake in the left condyle.

assessment can help determine the need for complex dental therapy. A study found 93% sensitivity and 86% specificity for scintigraphy as compared with 89% sensitivity and 27% specificity for tomography, in assessing TMJ pain and joint noise [29].

Bone scans aid in diagnosing conditions like TMJ disease, altering clinical diagnoses and treatment plans, and determining joint stability for dental rehabilitation, orthodontics, or orthognathic surgery. Negative scans indicate no active bony disease.

8.2 Single photon emission computed tomography (SPECT)

The TMJ is appropriate for single-photon emission CT (SPECT) scanning because it is a small joint located near the base of the skull and the paranasal sinuses. SPECT imaging allows for high-quality images of the TMJ that are separated from other high bone density regions, which planar images cannot do.

The TMJ can be investigated using one of the following techniques:

1. The 3-phase approach includes a 30-second perfusion study where images are obtained at every 3-seconds with computed perfusion analysis, instantaneous soft-tissue views of the head and mouth, and delayed views of the TMJ.

2. Delayed images include SPECT scans and planar views in anterior, posterior, and lateral projections of TMJ.

Increased perfusion and hyperemia are reflected in abnormal activity in TMJ flow studies in inflammatory individuals, with mild to substantial increases on immediate and delayed views (**Figure 19**). Being a non-anatomical examination is the main drawback of SPECT scanning. Although a region of elevated uptake indicating healing phenomena or aberrant pressures on the TMJ can be quickly established, the origin of these results may remain elusive.

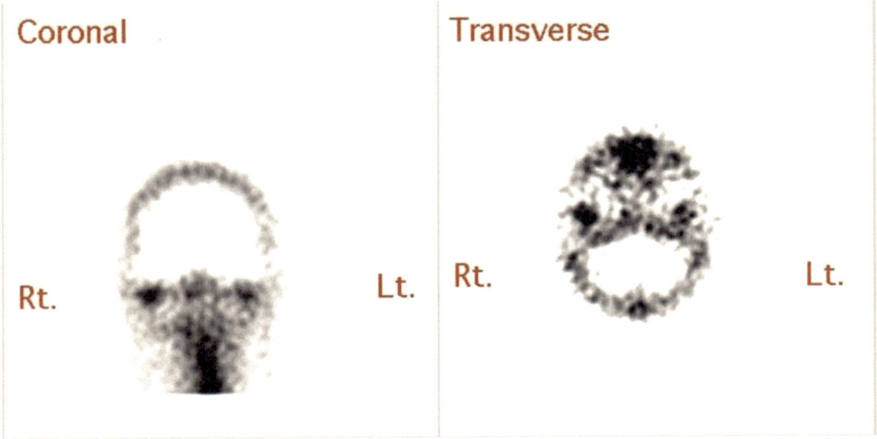

Figure 19.
Coronal and transaxial sections generated after single-photon emission computed tomography showing increased uptake in the right condyle.

SPECT using 99mTc MDP/HMDP is highly sensitive in detecting bone pathology, particularly TMJ meniscus abnormalities. Studies show a sensitivity of 68.75% and a specificity of 61.88%. Using SPECT scanning and semi-quantitative methods can improve results to 100% sensitivity and 83.33% specificity. Planar imaging can also detect additional lesions that resemble TMJ meniscus abnormalities and cause referred pain to the TMJ, such as upper cervical spine OA, bone metastases, and oral and sinus pathology. Although radionuclide imaging is highly sensitive, its specificity is low. Typically, any inflammatory/traumatic/neoplastic lesion exhibits enhanced isotope uptake, which is both advantageous and disadvantageous.

8.3 Positron emission tomography (PET)

Bone scans detect bone metabolic changes before structural changes, aiding early detection of TMD. However, due to a shortage of molybdenum-99, fluoride-18 positron emission tomography (18F-PET) is being considered for its superior sensitivity and image quality [30]. PET scans use a gamma camera and radiopharmaceuticals to detect metabolic processes. The most common radiopharmaceutical is 2-fluoro-2-deoxyglucose labeled with fluorine-18 (18FDG), which is up taken by areas with increased metabolism rates. PET-MRI is now used, combining CT, PET-CT, and MRI.

Patient preparation includes fasting for 6 hours, maintaining glucose level below 120mg/dl, hydration, and avoiding physical activity. PET scans should be performed 3 months post-surgery, which is up taken by areas with increased metabolism rates (**Figure 20**) [19, 31].

FDG-PET/CT has proven clinically useful in patients with TMD, osteoarthritis, and arthralgic TMJ and TMD osteoarthritis. Studies show high TMJ uptake ratios in patients with osteoarthritis, higher accuracy, and sensitivity compared to conventional bone scintigraphy. FDG PET's resolution for bone fractures is comparable to skeletal scintigraphy. PET scan evaluation requires thorough correlation with patient's medical history and other examinations, such as physical, laboratory, and diagnostic imaging. The mean effective dose for a PET scan is from 3 to 4 mSv (**Table 1**) [19].

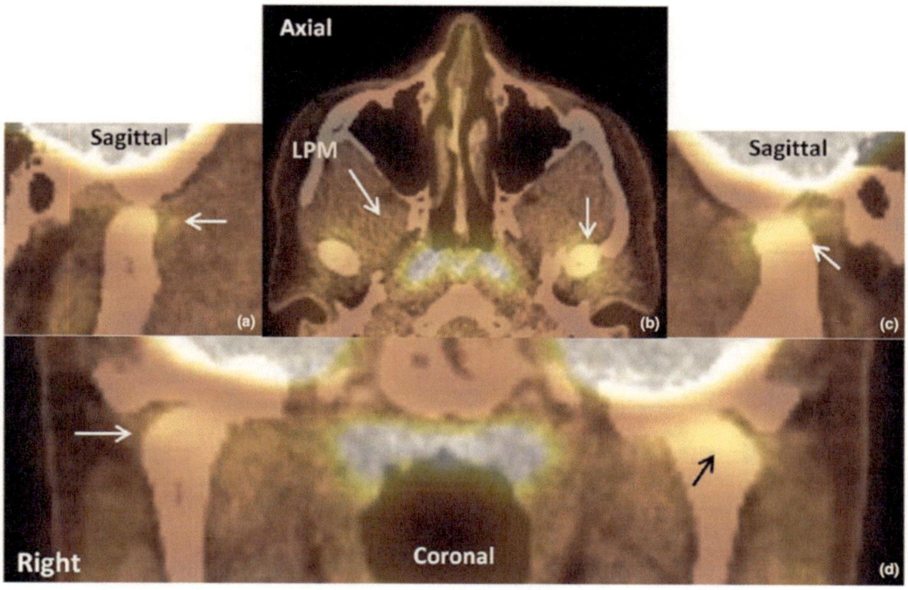

Figure 20.
Tempromandibular joint (TMJ) images obtained using positron emission tomography (PET). (a) Standard uptake value of the condylar head in sagittal view of the right TMJ. (b) Lateral pterygoid muscles and condyles seen in an axial view (LPM). (c) Sagittal image of the condyle and capsule in the left TMJ. (d) A coronal image showing the left and right TMJs. In RA-affected joints, inflammation (left >right) manifests as increased brightness. Increased brightness in the left condyle superiorly and laterally indicates increased absorption of 18-fluorodeoxyglucose (FDG). A comparison of the FDG uptake in the left and right condyle joints demonstrates the differences.

9. Radiographic appearance of TMJ disorders

TMJ pathology	Features	Imaging	
Dislocation/ Subluxation	Described as a condition in which the condyle moves excessively forward and beyond the articular eminence, completely separating the articular surfaces and fixing the condyle in place [19].	Diagnosis is primarily clinical. Panoramic radiograph (OPG) shows anterior and superior positioning of condyles to the articular eminence.	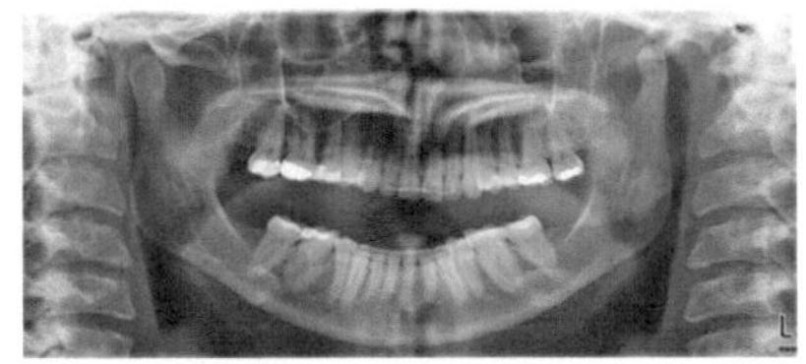 Panoramic radiograph showing anterior dislocation of left TMJ
Trauma/Intra-capsular fractures/ condylar fractures		OPG/3D CT scans provide sufficient information for treatment planning. The fractured fragments can be either medially or laterally displaced. Reduction of ramal height is also present. An open-mouth reverse Towne's view is ideal for detecting small fractures of the condyle that may not be seen on conventional radiography.	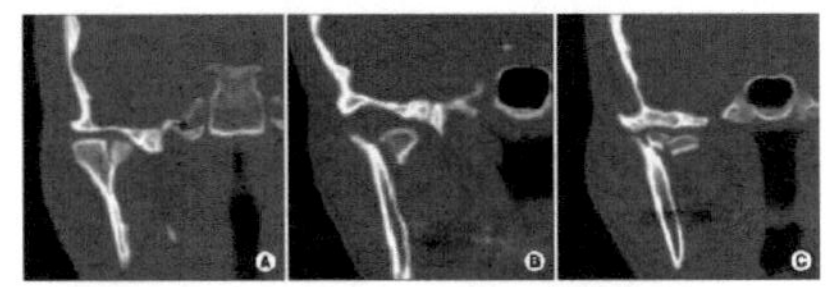 CT images showing intracapsular fractures 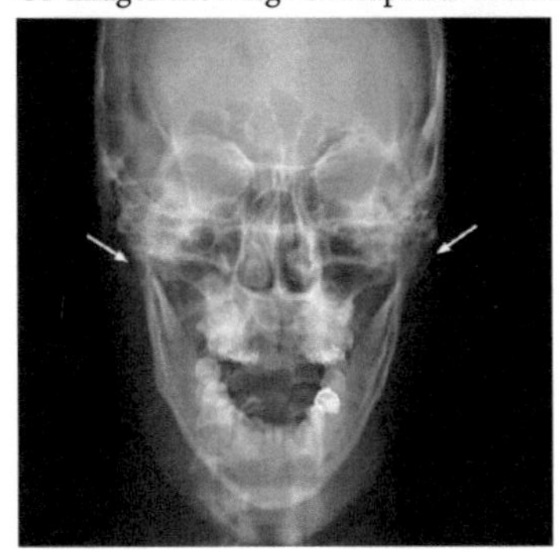 Reverse Town's view showing bilateral condylar fractures (arrows)

TMJ pathology	Features	Imaging	
Bifid Condyle	A bi-lobed or duplicated mandibular head, may be due to congenital fibrous septum, peripartum, or early childhood trauma, and may lie in antero-posterior or transverse orientation [8]. Missed malunited fractures may present as a bifid condyle	CT and MRI images may show bifid condyle as an incidental finding	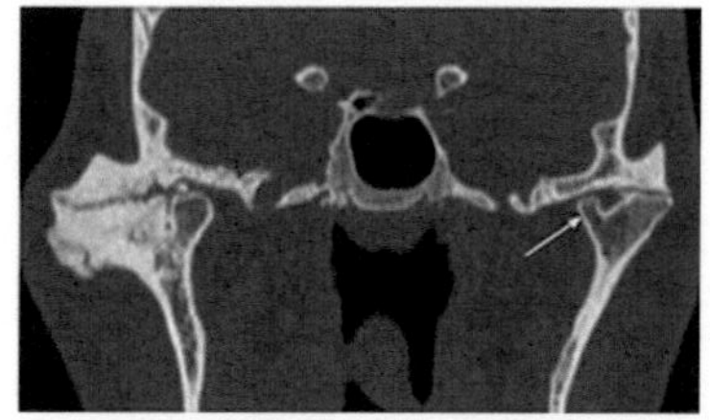 A coronal reconstructed computed tomography scan of the temporomandibular joint (TMJ) reveals a bifid left mandibular condyle. One of the condyles (arrow) is noticeably smaller than the other.
Condylar Agenesis/ Aplasia and Hypoplasia	The mandibular condyle can be partially or completely absent in a condylar deficiency. It can be the result of aberrant TMJ growth and development. Usually associated with hemifacial microsomia, Goldenhar syndrome, Treacher Collins syndrome, Proteus syndrome, Morquio syndrome, and auriculo-condylar syndrome	A short ramus and mandibular body, an undeveloped glenoid fossa, and a shallow sigmoid notch are all indicative of altered condylar form on CT and MRI scans.	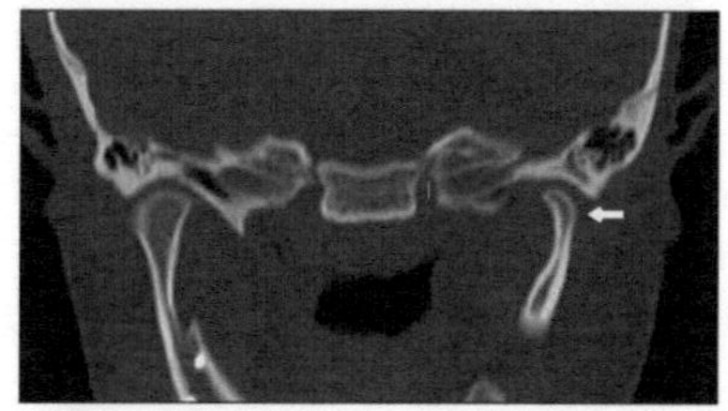 When compared to the normal right side, the coronal CT image in the bone window displays an underdeveloped left mandibular condyle and a shallow articular fossa.
Condylar Hyperplasia	Typically idiopathic, although it has been associated with endocrine disturbances	Radiological Signs of Affected Side: • Facial asymmetry. • Larger condylar head. • Normal or abnormal condylar head shape. • Increased mandible height. • Downward bowing of lower mandible border. • Lateral ramus bowing on postero-anterior radiographs.	

TMJ pathology	Features	Imaging	
			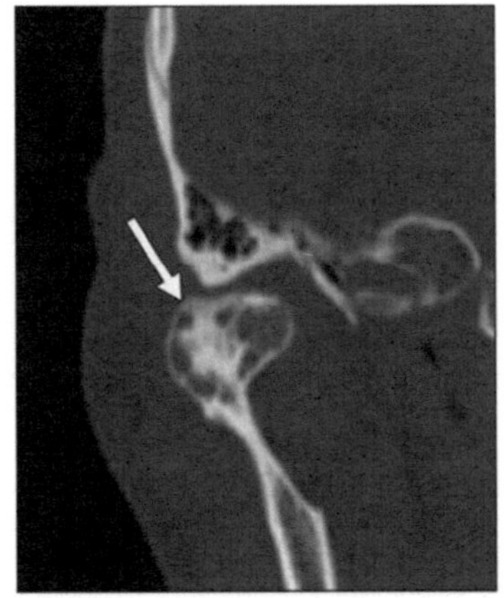 A coronal CT image obtained in the bone window reveals the mandibular condyle to be hyperplastic (arrow), impinging on the temporal bone next to it and lateral subluxation with respect to the articular fossa.
Condylar Resorption	Known as Cheerleader syndrome as most commonly affects teenage girls. It is a rapidly progressive condylar erosion resulting in widening of the joint space, which can be viewed in CT scan with the chin becoming less prominent as the disease progresses [8].	On radiographic or MRI examination, the volume of the condyle is diminished. The resorption generally occurs on the superior, antero-superior, or all other surfaces of the condylar head. This often results in an alteration of condylar contour. Bilateral anterior disc displacement with and without reduction are also seen. TMJ tomogram can be used as an alternative imaging modality [8].	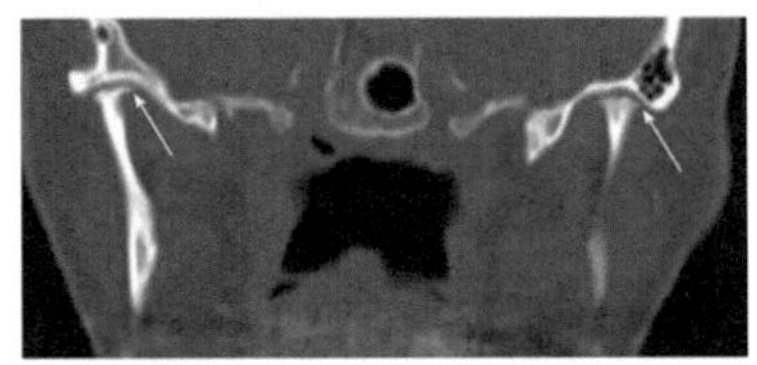 A young patient's temporomandibular joint shows a coronal reformatted computed tomography image with bilateral significant condylar resorption (arrows) but no signs of degenerative alterations within the joint.

DOI: http://dx.doi.org/10.5772/intechopen.1004930

TMJ pathology	Features	Imaging
Extensive pneumatization	Extensive pneumatization of the mastoid bone can involve the glenoid fossa and articular eminence. This information is especially necessary in TMJ surgical cases to prevent perforation and brain damage. Pneumatization also provides a pathway of least resistance for the spread of TMJ tumors [8].	CT must be performed prior to TMJ surgery when extensive pneumatization is detected in the panoramic radiographs [8] 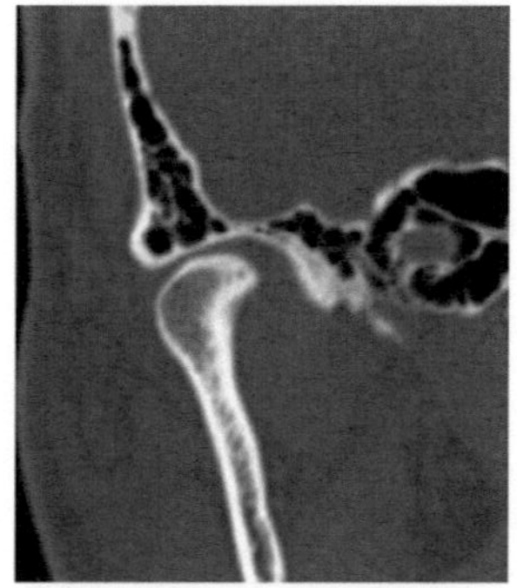 A coronal reconstructed computed tomography scan through the right temporomandibular joint shows nearly complete pneumatization of the glenoid fossa, with the exception of the central region.
Internal Derangement - Disk Displacement with Reduction	Defined as an abnormal anatomic relationship of the disk to the mandibular condyle. Causes include trauma, malocclusion, bruxism, stress, and primary osseous abnormalities [32]	MRI findings: anterior disk displacement in the closed-mouth view, with reduction in the open-mouth view; rounded or biconvex disk shape and abnormal disk position; increased T2 signal in the bilaminar zone; Loss of T1 and T2 signal is indicative of disk degeneration, as is an angle greater than 10° between the posterior band and the condyle's vertical orientation [32]. 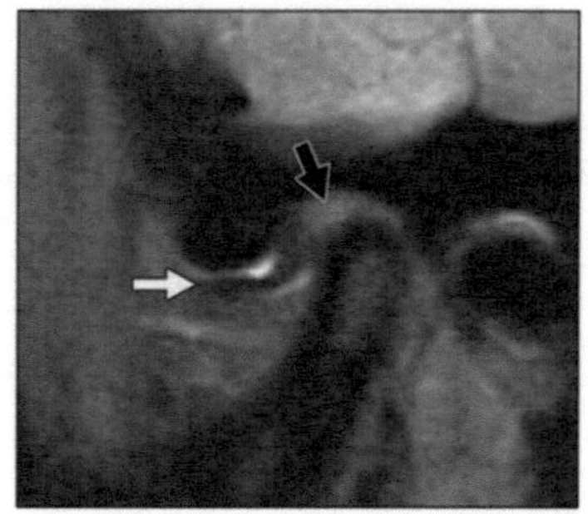 A The disk is anteriorly displaced, as seen in Sagittal closed-mouth proton density-weighted fat-saturated image (A) (white arrow). Additionally, the bilaminar zone exhibits an elevated T2 signal (black arrow), and the disk's typical shape is flattening.

TMJ pathology	Features	Imaging
		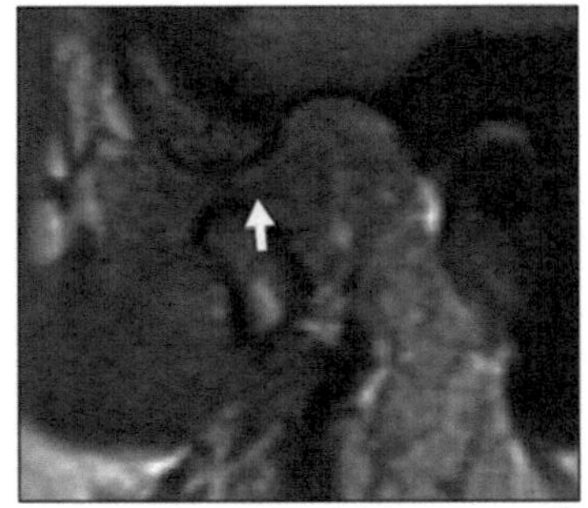 B The disk (arrow) decreases to its usual location in the sagittal open-mouth T1-weighted picture (B).
Internal Derangement - Disk Displacement without reduction	As the condition progresses, the posterior band thickens more and the anterior band mass decreases, leading to increasing laxity of the retrodiscal soft tissues and disk displacement without reduction. In more severe cases of internal disk derangement, a folded or flattened form is present [32].	MRI findings: low T2 signal in this area, suggesting fibrosis of a persistently displaced disk; high T2 signal of the retrodiscal tissues, suggesting inflammation and pain [32]

DOI: http://dx.doi.org/10.5772/intechopen.1004930

TMJ pathology	Features	Imaging
		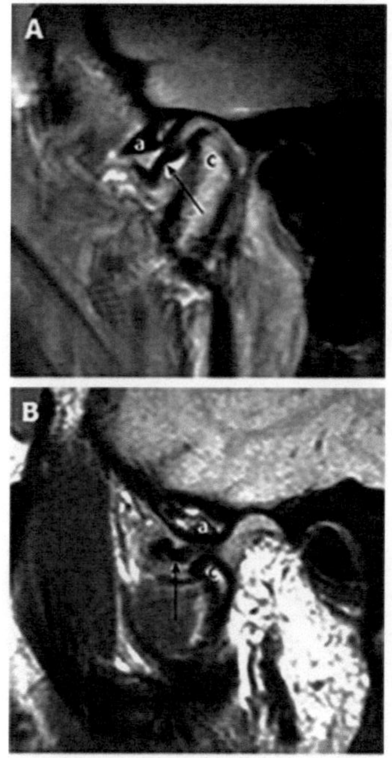 A: In closed mouth position, sagittal proton density weighted magnetic resonance imaging (MRI) shows anterior disk displacement (arrow), which is linked to the articular eminence (a) and anterior to the mandibular condyle (c). B: Open mouth sagittal proton density weighted MRI shows no decrease of the disk (arrow) between the mandibular condyle (c) and the articular eminence (a).

TMJ pathology	Features	Imaging
TMJ ankylosis	TMJ ankylosis can be caused by fibrous adhesions or a bone fusion, resulting in restricted jaw motion. Can occur as a sequel of previous infection, trauma, TMJ surgery, patients with juvenile idiopathic arthritis or bifid mandibular condyles [8].	MR arthrography is useful for the evaluation of fibrous adhesions and three-dimensional CT scan is necessary for surgical planning when bony fusion is suspected. Radiographic Findings: a. Orthopantomogra: i. Decreased joint space. ii. The absence or presence of typical condylar/coronoid anatomy. iii. A prominent antegonial notch. iv. Markings for osteotomy cuts for distraction. b. PA cephalogram: i. Chin deviation —Cg-ANS-Me (Crista Galli - Anterior Nasal Spine - Menton) ii. Occlusal cant iii. Grummon's analysis c. Lateral cephalogram: i. Ramal length: Ar-Go (Articulare-Gonion) ii. Corpus length: Go-Pog (Gonion-Pogonion) iii. Pharyngeal airway space (PAS) 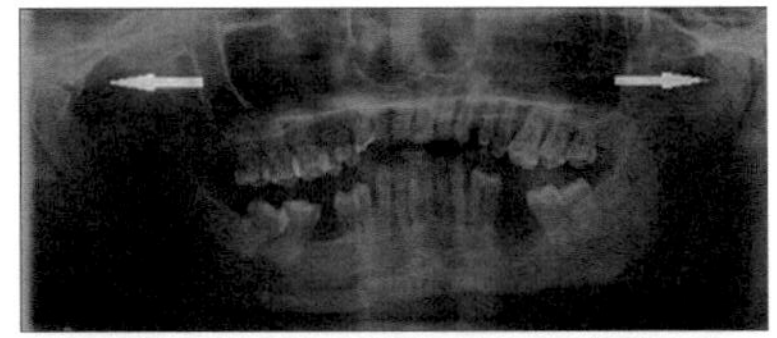 OPG showing loss of joint space (arrows) and a prominent antegonial notch. 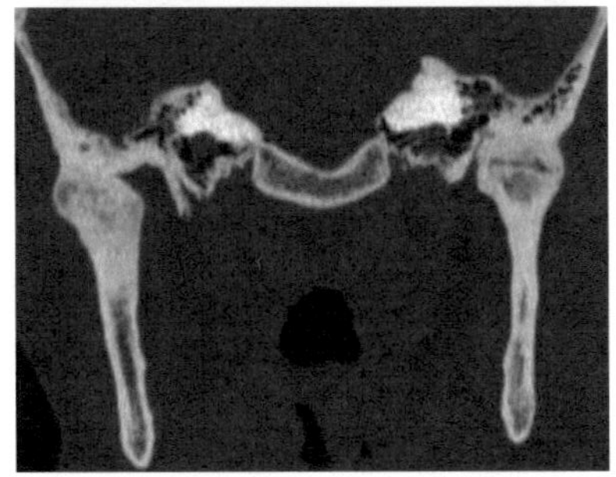 Coronal reconstruction of the axial dataset shows total ankylosis of the right temporomandibular joint (TMJ) and near-complete ankylosis of the left TMJ, with some residual joint space in the center (black arrow). 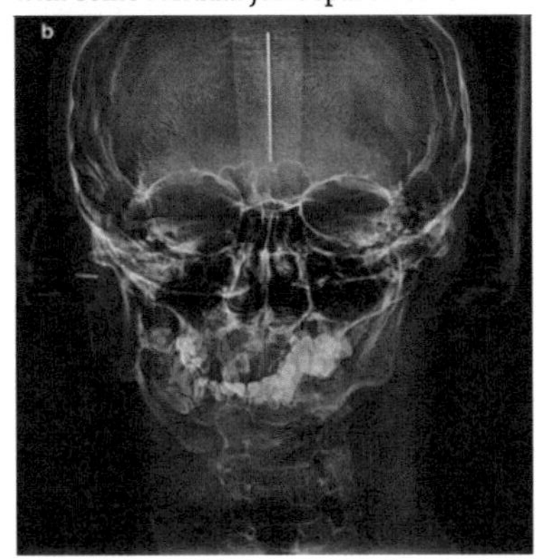 PA ceplalographic image showing deviation of chin towars the affected site along with presence of occlusal cant.

TMJ pathology	Features	Imaging
		iv. N perpendicular to Pog (Nasion perpendicular to Pogonion) d. Facial CT scan: i. Three-dimensional anatomy of bony morphology ii. Any necessary anatomical measures, such as the airway space volume, lingula position, ankylotic mass size, etc. e. CT Angiography CT Angiography may be essential to analyze the relationship between the internal maxillary artery and the ankylotic mass. There is a probability that the vessel is inside the bone, especially in re-ankylosis situations [33]. 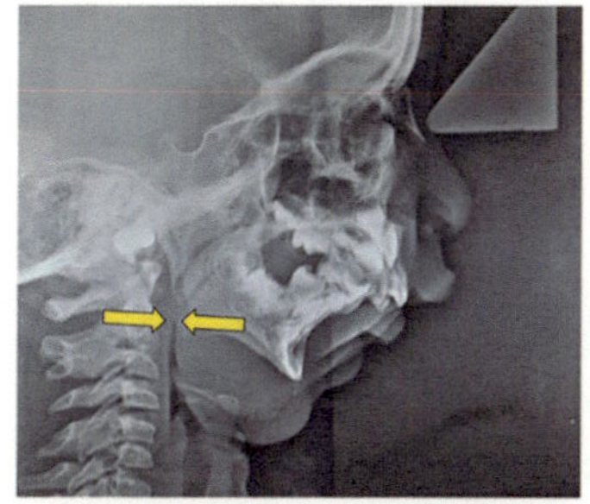 Lateral cephalogram shows decreased posterior airway space in case of bony ankylosis with a retruded chin. 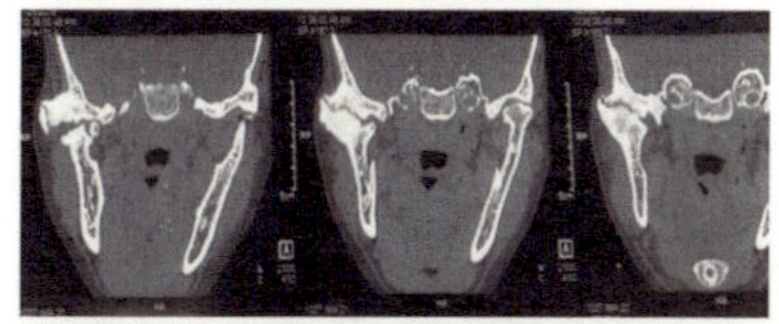 Coronal view of a CT scan showing right bony TMJ ankyloses. 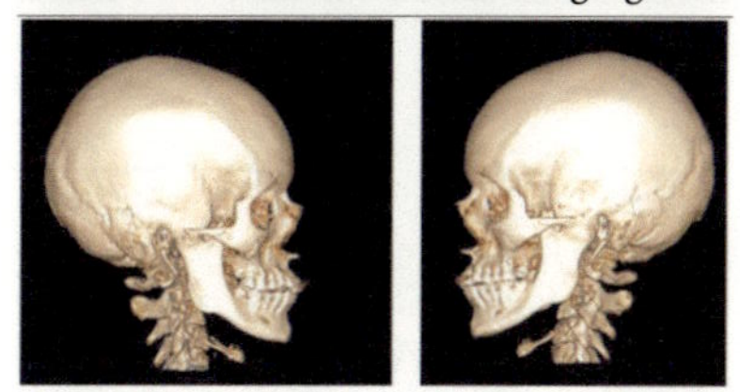 Pre-operative 3D reconstruction of CT scan images showing bilateral bony ankylosis of TMJ.

TMJ pathology	Features	Imaging	
			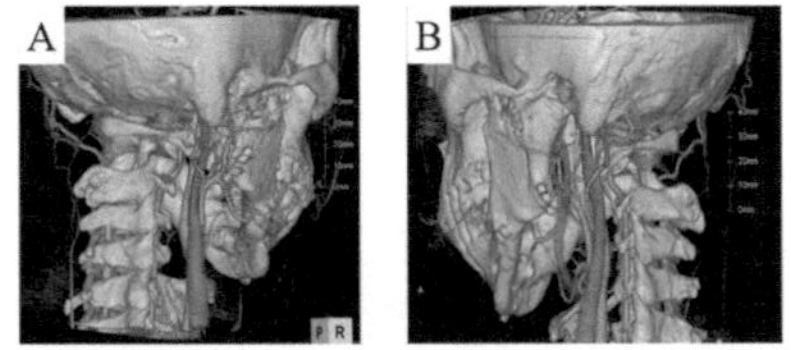 CT angiographic images shows close proximity of the maxillary artery bilaterally along the medial aspect of mandible as well as the bony ankylotic mass.
Benign/malignant neoplasms	a. Osteochondroma: It usually results in facial asymmetry, temporo-mandibular joint dysfunction, limited mouth opening and malocclusion. b. Chondrosarcoma: The clinical presentation typically refers to the most common pathologies like temporomandibular disorder, internal derangement, disc displacement, *degenerative joint disease*, which leads to diagnostic delay.	The Panoramic radiograph and open and close right TMJ views frequently shows a well-circumscribed oval-shaped mixed lesion having thin corticated rim. Varies from normal anatomy of condyle; usually presenting as condylar enlargement with or without lytic lesions associated. The precise location of the tumor and how it relates to the TMJ's anatomical features can be determined using MR and CT scans	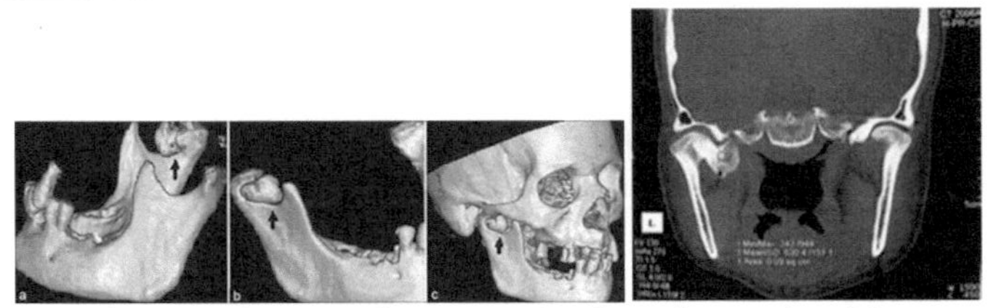 Coronal computed tomography cross section shows the margins of the osteochondroma. 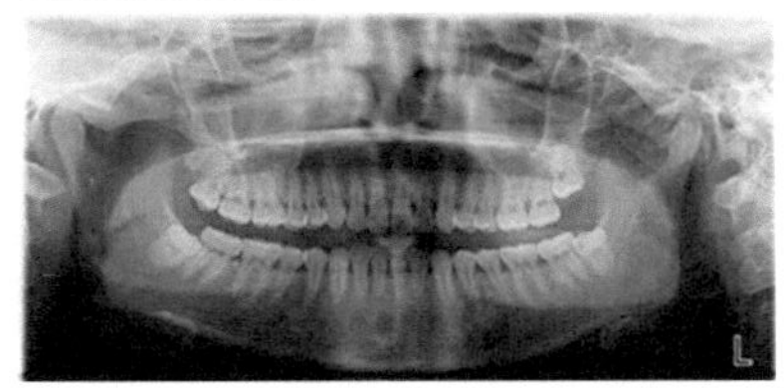 A panoramic radiograph of the patient reveals a radiopaque region on the left condylar region with the same density as the neighboring bone.

TMJ pathology	Features	Imaging
		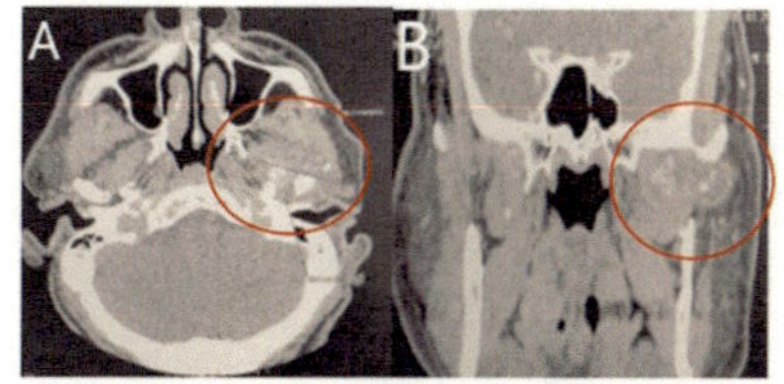 CT (Computed Tomography). A hypodense process with calcifications of 38 × 20 mm is localized on the left TMJ in both (A) axial and (B) coronal CT images with soft tissue setting. 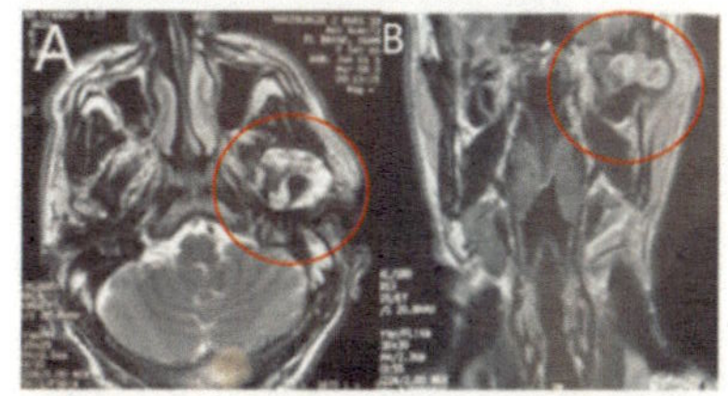 Magnetic resonance imaging (MRI) (A) Coronal and (B) axial views showed development at the left TMJ level. This creation measures 24.5 mm in height, 32.9 mm in diameter, and 43.1 mm in transverse diameter. It is seen in heterogeneous T2-weighted imaging (WI) high-intensity signals and low-intensity signals T1-WI. There is no mandibular bone anomaly in contrast to a 9 mm bone discontinuity around the base of the skull.

TMJ pathology	Features	Imaging
TMJ arthritis	i. Inflammatory arthritis: 1. *Juvenile idiopathic arthritis* (JIA) is the most prevalent rheumatic illness in children, affects girls more often than boys. Synovial joints are primarily affected by the condition. 2. *Rheumatoid arthritis (RA)* is a chronic inflammatory condition that mostly affects the tissue around the joints, including the ligaments, synovial membrane, joint capsules, and tendons. Internal joint components play a secondary role. ii. Degenerative arthritis: 1. *Osteoarthritis (OA)* is most commonly involving pathology of TMJ which is a chronic degenerative disease that characteristically affects the articular cartilage of synovial joints and is associated with simultaneous remodeling of the	OPG, CT, MRI and ultrasound have been used to evaluate TMJ JIA. OPG and CT are most effective at detecting bone erosions caused by TMJ involvement. USG and MRI has better soft tissue resolution for earlier diagnosis. Condylar resorption can be better evaluated on non-fat suppressed T1 weighted sequence and suggests a more chronic TMJ arthritis. Loss of joint space, condylar destruction, flattening with anterior positioning of the condyle. There may be flattening of the articular eminence and erosion of the glenoid fossa. Synovial proliferation is an early phase in RA that distinguishes it from other forms of arthritis. Synovial proliferation is visible on MRI and can occur in all patients [32]. CT scans reveal calcium accumulation in the disk or periarticular tissue. CPP deposits often present as hypointense material on both T1 and T2 weighted MRI scans [32].

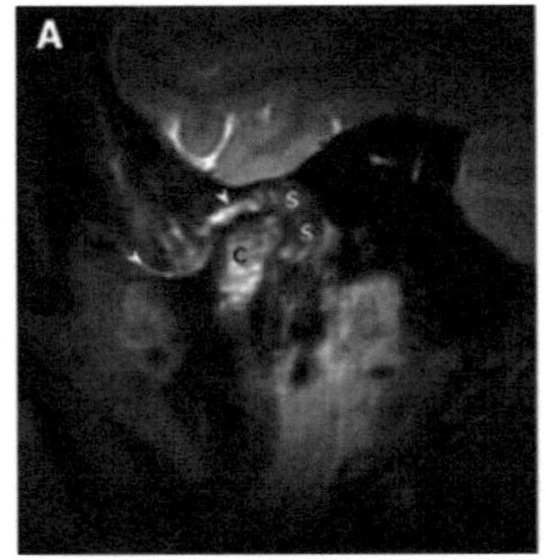

A. Sagittal proton density weighted magnetic resonance imaging (MRI) in the closed mouth position reveals enhanced signal at the mandibular condyle (c) and synovial thickening (s) in the retrodiscal areas. Thickening and enhanced signal of the synovium in various areas (arrowheads).

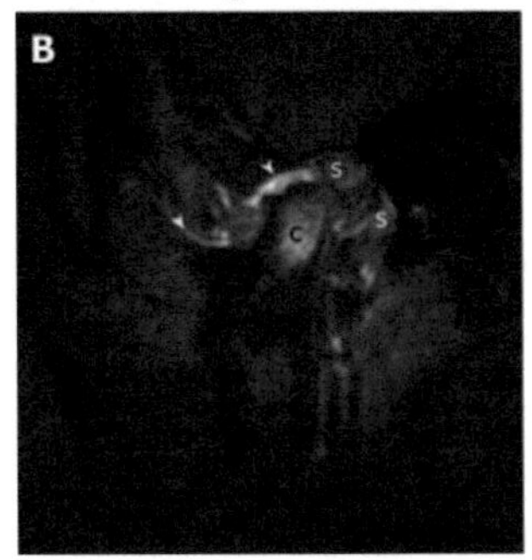

B. Sagittal fat suppressed post contrast T1 weighted MRI in the closed mouth position demonstrates enhancement of signal at the mandibular condyle (c), enhancement and extensive thickening of the synovium (s) in the retrodiscal regions. Thickening and enhancement of the synovium at other places as well (arrowheads).

TMJ pathology	Features	Imaging
	underlying subchondral bone with secondary involvement of the synovium [32] 2. Metabolic arthritis: *Calcium pyrophosphate dehydrate deposition disease (CPPD):* is a metabolic arthropathy characterized by the deposition of calcium pyrophosphate dehydrate crystals in and around joints, particularly the articular cartilage and fibrocartilage [32].	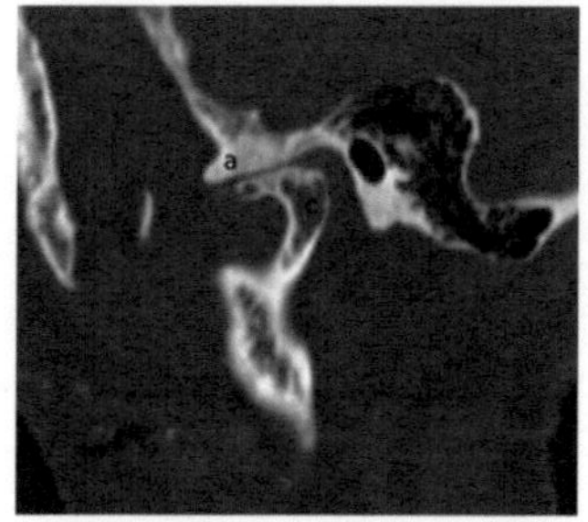 C. Sagittal reformation of the axial dataset shows deformation of the mandibular condyle (c), significant sclerosis of the articular eminence (a), and severe loss of joint space. 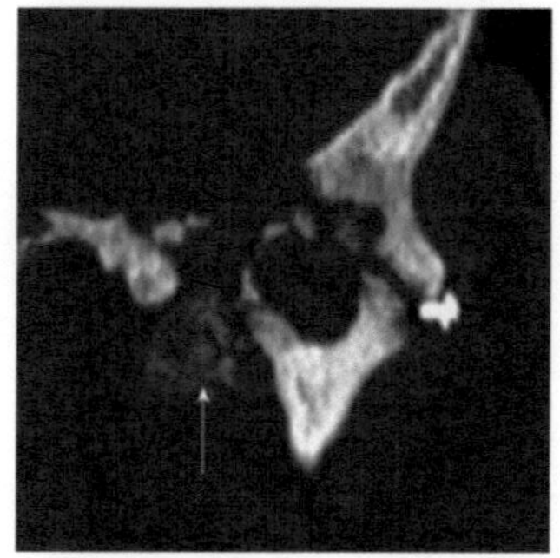 D. Coronal reformation of the axial dataset shows that the left temporomandibular joint has been destroyed, with erosion and distortion of both the mandibular condyle and the glenoid fossa. There is widespread calcium pyrophosphate dehydrate deposition illness at the joint space (arrow).

Table 1.
Depicting the clinical and radiographic features of various TMJ disorders/pathology.

Author details

Neha Nainoor* and Gunjan Pani
Consultant Oral and Maxillofacial Surgeon, Department of Oral and Maxillofacial Surgery, Rajiv Gandhi University of Health Sciences, Bangalore, Karnataka, India

*Address all correspondence to: drnehanomfs@gmail.com

References

[1] Aiken A, Bouloux G, Hudgins P. MR imaging of the temporomandibular joint. Magnetic Resonance Imaging Clinics of North America. 2012;**20**:397-412. DOI: 10.1016/j.mric.2012.05.002, 10.1016/j.mric.2012.05.002

[2] Guralnick W, Kaban LB, Merrill RG. Temporomandibular-joint afflictions. The New England Journal of Medicine. 1978;**299**:123-129. DOI: 10.1056/NEJM197807202990304

[3] Gatchel RJ, Stowell AW, Wildenstein L, Riggs R, Ellis E 3rd. Efficacy of an early intervention for patients with acute temporomandibular disorder related pain: A one-year outcome study. Journal of the American Dental Association (1939). 2006;**137**(3):339-347

[4] de Senna BR, dos Santos Silva VK, França JP, Marques LS, Pereira LJ. Imaging diagnosis of the temporomandibular joint: Critical review of indications and new perspectives. Oral Radiology. 2009;**25**:86-98

[5] Gupta A, Jain D, Sampath S. Conventional and contemporary diagnostic tools in temporomandibular disorders–an overview. International Journal. 2020;**3**:716

[6] Scarfe WC, Farman AG, Sukovic P. Clinical applications of cone-beam computed tomography in dental practice. Journal of the Canadian Dental Association. 2006;**72**(1):75-80

[7] Marques AP, Perrella A, Arita ES, Pereira MF, Cavalcanti MG. Assessment of simulated mandibular condyle bone lesions by cone beam computed tomography. Brazilian Oral Research. 2010;**24**(4):467-474

[8] Bag AK, Gaddikeri S, Singhal A, Hardin S, Tran BD, Medina JA, et al. Imaging of the temporomandibular joint: An update. World Journal of Radiology. 2014;**6**(8):567

[9] White SC, Pharoah MJ. Textbook of Oral Radiology Principles and Interpretation. 6th ed. St. Louis, Missouri: Mosby Elsevier Publisher; 2010

[10] Karjodkar F. Textbook of Dental and Maxillofacial Radiology. 2nd ed. Daryaganj, New Delhi, India: Jaypee Brothers Medical Publishers (P) Ltd.; 2009

[11] Whates E. Essentials of Dental Radiography and Radiology. 3rd ed. Philadelphia, USA: Elsevier's Health Sciences Rights Department; 2002

[12] Dhabale GS, Bhowate RR. Cone-beam computed tomography for temporomandibular joint imaging. Cureus. 2022;**14**(11):e31515. DOI: 10.7759/cureus.31515

[13] Barghan S, Tetradis S, Mallya SM. Application of cone beam computed tomography for assessment of the temporomandibular joints. Australian Dental Journal. 2012;**57**:109-118

[14] Boeddinghaus R, Whyte A. CT of the TMJ. Journal of Medical Imaging and Radiation Oncology. 2013;**57**:448-454. DOI: 10.1111/1754-9485.12021

[15] Pahwa S, Bhalla AS, Roychaudhary A, Bhutia O. Multidetector computed tomography of temporomandibular joint: A road less travelled. World Journal of Clinical Cases. 2015;**3**(5):442-449. DOI: 10.12998/wjcc.v3.i5.442

[16] Larheim T, Abrahamsson A-k, Kristensen M, Arvidsson L. Temporomandibular joint diagnostics using CBCT. Dento Maxillo Facial Radiology. 2014;**44**:20140235. DOI: 10.1259/dmfr.20140235

[17] Caruso S, Storti E, Nota A, Ehsani S, Gatto R. Temporomandibular joint anatomy assessed by CBCT images. BioMed Research International. 2017; **2017**:2916953

[18] Juárez VP. Diagnostic efficacy of cone beam computed tomography for the TMJ arthropathies. Journal of Dental Health, Oral Disorders & Therapy. 2020; **11**(6):176-185. DOI: 10.15406/jdhodt.2020.11.00538

[19] Różyło-Kalinowska I. Nuclear medicine in TMJ imaging. In: Rozylo-Kalinowska I, Orhan K, editors. Imaging of the Temporomandibular Joint. Cham: Springer; 2019. DOI: 10.1007/978-3-319-99468-0_12

[20] Yadav KD, Prasad RS, Raghunand SJ, Mohammed S, Anuradha P. TMJ arthrography. International journal of maxillofacial Imaging. 2019;**5**(1):1-2

[21] Levring Jäghagen E, Ahlqvist J. Arthrography of the temporomandibular joint: Main diagnostic and therapeutic applications. Clinical and Experimental Dental Research. 2020;**4**:2. DOI: 10.1007/s41894-019-0064-6

[22] Surej Kumar LK, Zachariah GP, Chandran S. Ultrasonography: A step forward in temporomandibular joint imaging. A preliminary descriptive study. Clinics and Practice. 2019;**9**(2): 1134. DOI: 10.4081/cp.2019.1134

[23] Maranini B, Ciancio G, Mandrioli S, Galiè M, Govoni M. The role of ultrasound in temporomandibular joint disorders: An update and future perspectives. Frontiers in Medicine. 2022;**9**:926573. DOI: 10.3389/fmed.2022.926573

[24] Emshoff R, Bertram S, Rudisch A, Gassner R. The diagnostic value of ultrasonography to determine the temporomandibular joint disk position. Oral Surgery, Oral Medicine, Oral Pathology, Oral Radiology, and Endodontics. 1997;**84**:688-696. DOI: 10.1016/S1079-2104(97)90374-7

[25] Jank S, Haase S, Strobl H, Michels H, Hafner R, Missmann M, et al. Sonographic investigation of the temporomandibular joint in patients with juvenile idiopathic arthritis: A pilot study. Arthritis and Rheumatism. 2007; **57**:213-218. DOI: 10.1002/art.22533

[26] Malusare PC et al. Advanced TMJ imaging-a review. Clinical Radiology and Imaging Journal. 2019;**3**(4):000153

[27] Baba IA, Najmuddin M, Shah AF, Yousuf A. TMJ imaging: A review. International Journal of Contemporary Medical Research. 2016;**3**(8):2253-2256

[28] Lee YH, Hong IK, Chun YH. Prediction of painful temporomandibular joint osteoarthritis in juvenile patients using bone scintigraphy. Clinical and Experimental Dental Research. 2019;**5**(3):225-235. DOI: 10.1002/cre2.175

[29] Epstein JB, Rea A, Chahal O. The use of bone scintigraphy in temporomandibular joint disorders. Oral Diseases. 2002;**8**(1):47-53

[30] Lee JW, Lee SM, Kim SJ, Choi JW, Baek KW. Clinical utility of fluoride-18 positron emission tomography/CT in temporomandibular disorder with osteoarthritis: Comparisons with 99mTc-MDP bone scan. Dento Maxillo Facial

Radiology. 2013;**42**(2):29292350. DOI: 10.1259/dmfr/29292350

[31] Rice DD, Abramovitch K, Roche S, Cora CA, Torralba KD, Christensen HL, Christiansen EL. Undiagnosed, chronic temporomandibular joint pain: Making a case for FDG-PET/CT. International Journal of Rheumatic Diseases. 2017;**20**(12):2122-2126. DOI: 10.1111/1756-185X.13134

[32] Petscavage-Thomas JM, Walker EA. Unlocking the jaw: Advanced imaging of the temporomandibular joint. American Journal of Roentgenology. 2014;**203**(5): 1047-1058

[33] Anchlia S. Temporomandibular joint ankylosis. In: Bonanthaya K, Panneerselvam E, Manuel S, Kumar VV, Rai A, editors. Oral and Maxillofacial Surgery for the Clinician. Singapore: Springer; 2021. DOI: 10.1007/978-981-15-1346-6_65

Chapter 2

Diagnosis and Treatment of Myofascial Pain Syndrome in Temporomandibular Dysfunction

Leandro Díez-Suárez, Rodrigo Garay Symor and Arturo Ivan Espinosa Carlos

Abstract

The temporomandibular joint (TMJ) is an important structure of the facial skeleton and is an important source of pain when inflammatory processes are occurring in it. It is located inferior the skull base, above the neck and anterior to the ear. The principal components include: bone structures, ligaments, intrarticular content, and muscles. Because of the anatomic relations, the temporomandibular joint affections can produce a limitation of the masticatory function and express headache of dental, sinusal, nervous, or muscular type. For this reason, the patients require multiple medical and dental specialties in the search of a solution for the current illness. The myofascial pain refers to a chronic, inflammatory condition of the TMJ and the muscular system of the head and neck. It has an important demand in the health sector, can incapacitate significantly the quality of life of the patients, and requires an appropriate diagnosis and treatment. The aim of this chapter is to guide the clinical practice in the etiology, diagnosis, prevention, and treatment of the myofascial pain as a clinical presentation of the temporomandibular dysfunction.

Keywords: myofascial pain, trigger point, TMJ dysfunction, referred pain, botulinum toxin

1. Introduction

The temporomandibular joint "TMJ" is a ginglymoid, arthrodial, and compounded joint. It presents an articular biconcave disk that is interposed between the temporal and mandibular bone. It is located inferior the skull base, above the neck, anterior to the ear, and behind the ear. Its anatomical structures of relevance are divided in 4 big components: bone structures, ligaments, intrarticular components, and muscles [1].

Because of the masticatory function, TMJ has an important muscular component. The main muscles related to the masticatory function and the TMJ are the temporal, masseter, medial pterygoid, and lateral pterygoid. Nevertheless, there is a wide muscular network that extends from the head, neck, and upper back that could be affected in articular dysfunction presentations [2].

The temporomandibular dysfunction refers to a group of disorders that affect the TMJ; this affections can have an origin such as anatomic, growth and development, tumoral, traumatic, systemic disease, and acute or chronic inflammatory conditions, among others [3, 4].

It is estimated that more than 5% of the population presents some type of temporomandibular dysfunction, and a 6–12% of the general population could have a sign or symptom suggestive of TMD [2]. Generally, the temporomandibular dysfunction is presented in 2/3 of the feminine population, between 20 and 40 years of age, and exists an antecedent that triggers the symptomatology in the patients such as recent dental treatments, anxiety, depression, and tension type conditions, among others [2, 5]. Although the temporomandibular dysfunction could present signs and symptoms at early ages, the myofascial pain is often diagnosed at an older age. This is because the psychosocial triggers appear at an elderly age and the patients usually consult when the symptomatology has years of evolution.

Myofascial pain síndrome (MPS) is a chronic condition of dysfunction and inflammatory joint with multifactorial etiology that located the pain in the head and neck region [6].

Because of the anatomic relation, a lot of patients with TMJ dysfunction require health services, which can involve specialists such as neurologists, otolaryngologists, pain medicine, rheumatologists, physiotherapists, and dentists [7]. This pain can stimulate other conditions in the head and neck, so the diagnosis is very important to bring an adequate attention to patients with TMJ dysfunction [8].

2. Diagnostic of the myofascial pain syndrome

The main symptom of the patients with joint dysfunction is the pain and the most difficult to evaluate. The pain in the temporomandibular region could appear in different ways. An electric, burning, or searing type of pain refers to disorders of nervous of neuralgic type. The auriculotemporal nerve is the principal nerve of the TMJ. The compression of the auriculotemporal nerve may be due a disk displacement or an anatomical variation of the joint [8].

A deep, dull, irradiated, and not located pain frequently relates with a muscular disorder. The myalgia refers as a muscle band that suffered an inflammatory process (trigger point) that radiates the pain [9].

The main challenge for the clinician is to establish the origin of the pain. Detailing if the pain has a dental, articular, nervous, or muscular origin could be difficult. The anesthetic blockade is a useful tool to differentiate from a dental, neuralgic, or muscular pain [10].

The anesthetic blockade can be done for a tooth or a group of teeth on a regular basis so that you can exclude a possible dental cause.

The anesthetic blockade of the auriculotemporal nerve can be done by placing the needle behind the neck of the condylar process to the posterior aspect of the mandibular ramus. The patient can open and close the mouth, so you can feel the position of the needle on the bone and place 0.5 ml of 1% simple lidocaine [11].

The aim of the anesthetic blockade is to differentiate the articular pain such as capsulitis, synovitis, or any neuropathic pain of the myofascial pain (**Figure 1**).

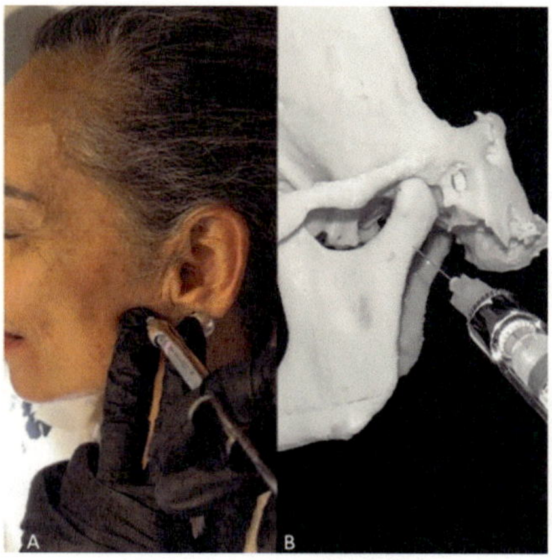

Figure 1.
A. Anesthetic block of the auriculotemporal nerve. B. Anatomical reference.

2.1 Medical history and e interrogatory

The information about the beginning and type of pain is fundamental to achieve an adequate diagnosis. The health questionnaire has to include questions addressed to systemic diseases that could be related to the myofascial pain or joint dysfunction. Because the TMJ is a synovial joint, the disorders that affect other joints could affect the TMJ. Interrogating the patient about another symptom of other joints of the body could relate an autoimmune affection or a rheumatoid systemic condition. The main illnesses that affect the joint system are fibromyalgia, rheumatoid arthritis, and others [2].

72% patients with joint dysfunction and myofascial pain can have ear symptomatology. It is important to investigate about symptoms such as vertigo, dizziness, sensation of plugged ear, tinnitus, or ear pain [12].

The pain is the main symptom that patients refer and has lots of presentations. A pain that appears in the morning or when they wake up could be related with bruxism. A pain that appears ending the day could be related to tensional conditions or stress. On many occasions, the psychological and emotional condition of the patients could affect the muscular system and the sleep cycle producing tensional states. Generally, mourning, unemployment, or anxious or depressive personal situations could trigger a muscular painful condition [13, 14].

2.2 Articular exam

A healthy temporomandibular joint has a mouth opening between 35 to 60 mm, but this measure can vary from age to age; movements of opening that are increased (hypermobility) could be related to an hyperlaxity of the ligaments, a flat and joint and a condilar luxation or subluxation. In contrast, a reduced opening (hypomobility) could be related to a degradation and entrapment of the articular disk or active inflammatory processes [15].

Deviation, clicking, and joint sounds can show a bone asymmetry with chronic deterioration and degenerative of the articular disk, but this is part of another chapter. However, the integral examination has to include palpation, auscultation, and the registration of deviations at the opening or closure of the mandible [16].

2.3 Muscular exam

The muscular exam of the head and neck must be exhaustive and as important as the others for the diagnosis of the myofascial pain.

The first step before the initial exam is to educate the patient in order to determine the level of pain. Under a visual analogue scale (VAS) of the pain, the patient can refer when the pain is mild (1–3 points), moderate (4–6 points), or severe (7–10 points) (**Figure 2**).

The second step is to guide the patient to identify the most painful palpation zone, if the pain radiates behind another anatomical structure of the head or neck (e.g., eyes, periorbital area, frown, head, neck, back of the neck, shoulders, teeth, etc.).

The third step is to begin the exploration of the musculature of the head and neck in an orderly way. The professional stands behind the head of the patient and mak-ing a bilateral exploration. Attention must be paid to the gestures that the patient does when the palpation is applied. Many patients present a high threshold, even if they qualified the pain as mild; this could be moderate or severe (**Figure 3**). Some patients, even if they present a high threshold, express a palpebral reaction or a departure with severe pain [2].

The palpation strength has to be steady, oriented, and local. Some muscles show multiple fascicles, and these must be palpated. It is needed an adequate anatomical study of the zone, to identify correctly the origin, insertion, and the layout of the fibers of every muscle. In this manner, we can identify the trigger points and the hypertrophic and symptomatic muscle bands.

Care should be taken to the blood vessels of the neck region, for not generating a vasopressor effect. In the intraoral region, the muscular band and the referred pain must be identified properly in order to differentiate neuropathic pain with radiate pain [9].

2.4 Intraoral exam

The intraoral exam consists of several points; it must include the dental analysis, demonstrating the health or illness of any dental organ, through a meticulous examination of the dental arches, dental position, and evaluation of Spee and Wilson curves. Percussion tests must be done with the suggesting dental organs to present any associated pathology.

Evaluating the dental position is important for the diagnosis, because it can guide the clinician to the existence of an imbalance between dental arches; this can be done with a previous interrogatory about the stability perceived from the patient when eating, swallowing, and so forth, with the colocation of dental paper, to verify the presence of any premature contact points and if there is any midline discrepancy or differences between the molar relationship [17].

As a complement to the muscular examination, in the intraoral examination, we must palpate the lateral pterygoid muscles. To achieve this, we must direct palpation towards the infratemporal fossa [2].

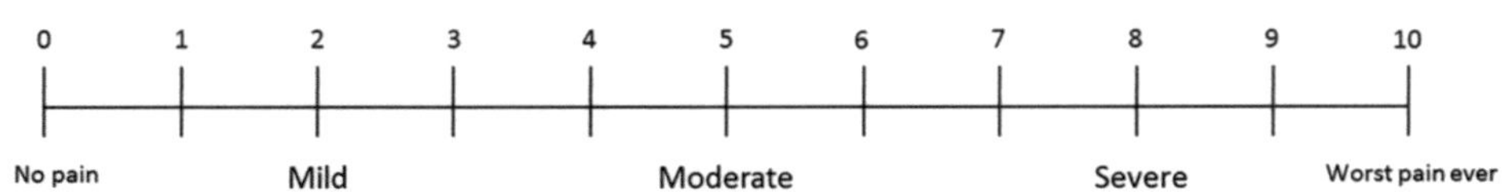

Figure 2.
Visual analog scale used for all of our patients.

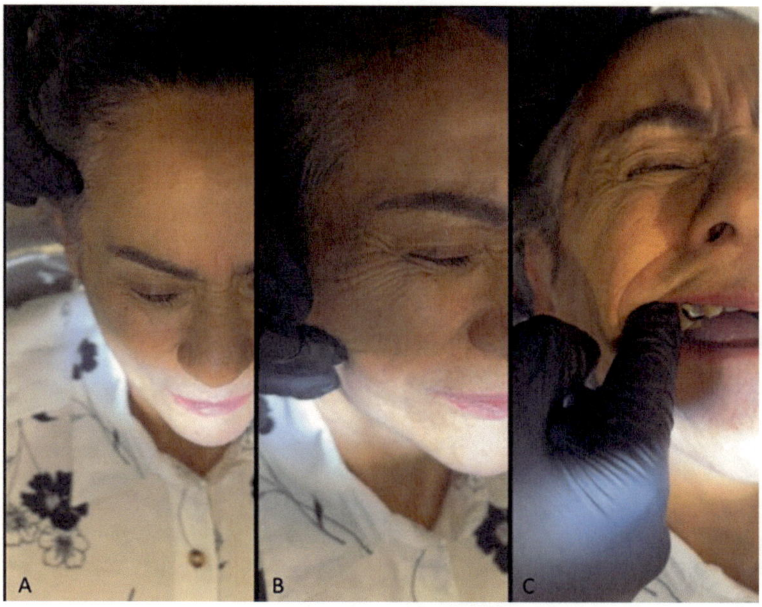

Figure 3.
Head and neck muscle examination: A. Temporal muscle. B. Masseter muscle. C. Lateral pterygoid muscle.

2.5 Imaging studies

The use of imaging studies is very useful to complete the diagnosis. The periapical radiographs are helpful to determine the origin of dental pain or any other pathologies. The cone-beam computed tomography scans and the panoramic radiographs can provide better details about the bone and joint structures of the TMJ, but not the articular disk (**Figure 4**). However, MRI could be considered as the best option to evaluate the articular disk; it allows to see the position, morphology, and degenerative changes of the bones [2].

3. Myofascial pain syndrome treatment

The MPS treatment is complex; there are different initiators or trigger factors. As already mentioned, MPS is composed of peripheral inflammatory processes with a huge psychosocial compound.

The treatment must have an integral and multidisciplinary focus. Particularly at a muscular level, the treatment must be addressed in the muscular trigger points, seeking to correct the structural and muscular imbalance. This can be done through different actions, such as pharmacologic strategies, physical therapy, and intraoral devices, among others [6, 18].

3.1 Pharmacological management

Because of the multifactorial nature of the myofascial pain syndrome (MPS), it can appear with an insidious, trauma, or injury onset [6]. There will be a release of inflammatory mediators that sensitize the peripheral nociceptors [19]. Actually, it can develop a "central sensitization" it consists of an amplified response of the

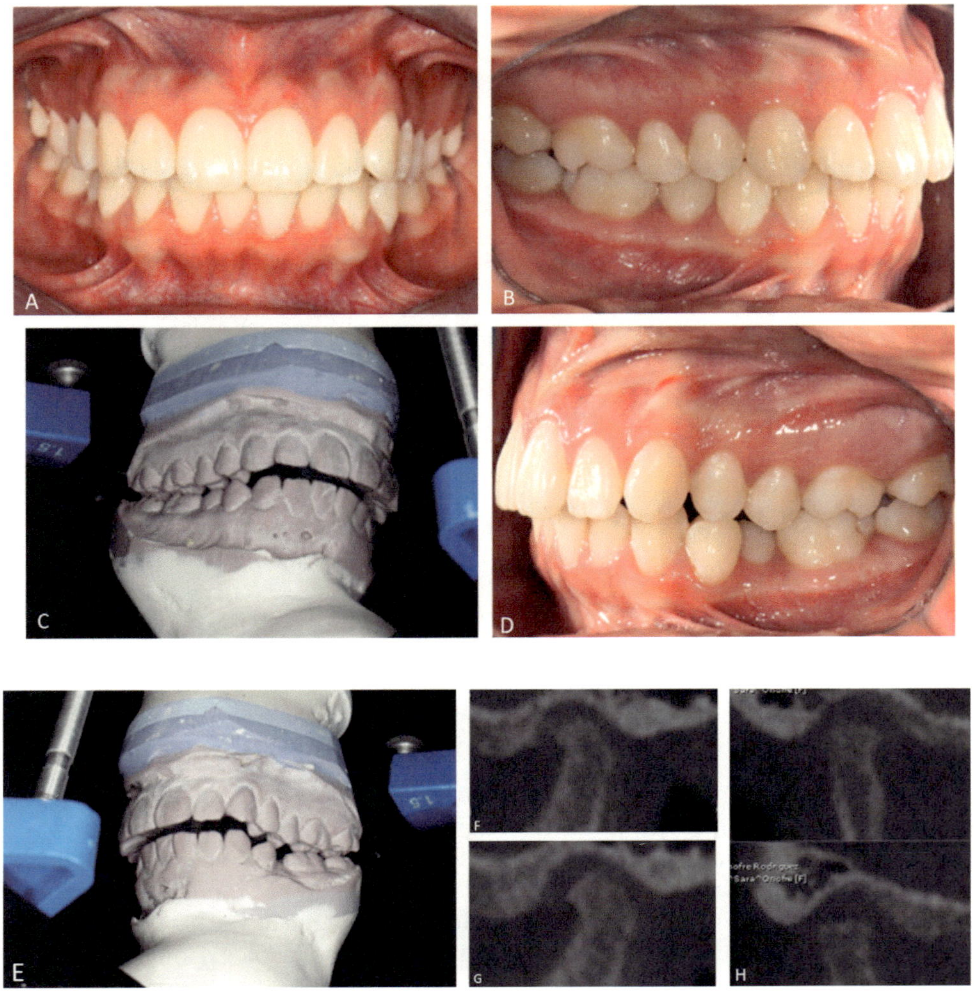

Figure 4.
A–E. Occlusion with diagnostic mounting. F–H. TC scan (note the irregularity of the cortical bone of the mandibular condyle).

CNS, characterized for a hyperexcitability of the neurons of the dorsal spinal horns, causing hypersensitivity and/or allodynia. This response is present in patients with MPS; that is why you should seek pharmacological treatment to reduce it [20].

3.1.1 Nonsteroidal anti-inflammatory drugs (NSAIDs)

These drugs inhibit the cyclooxygenase (COX) 1 and 2 blocking the prostaglandins synthesis; this reduces the sensitization and excitation of the peripheral nociceptors [21].

It is important to say COX-1 is present in most of the tissues; it participates in the formation of relevant prostaglandins (PG) to regulate the hemostasis, kidney integrity, platelet function, protection of gastric mucosa (PG12), and so on. Meanwhile, COX-2 is inducible especially in inflammatory processes [21, 22].

3.1.2 NSAIDs classification

The NSAIDs are divided in 3 groups depending on their selectivity to the inhibition of COX-2, such as Nonselective (Aspirin, Diflunisal, Ibuprofen, Ketoprofen, Naproxen, Meclofenamate, and Piroxicam), Semiselective or preferential to COX-2 (Diclofenac, Etodolac, and Meloxicam), and Highly Selective (Celecoxib, Etoricoxib, Lumiracoxib, Rofecoxib, and Valdecoxib) [23].

Also, these drugs can be classified depending on their chemical structure, such as derived from salicylic acid (acetylsalicylic, nonselective but very aggressive with gastric mucosa), aryl-propionic (Ibuprofen and naproxen, nonselective), acetic acid (diclofenac and ketorolac) and anthranilic acid (both are hematologically toxic), enolic acid or oxicams (piroxicam, tenoxicam, and meloxicam, the last one is preferential to COX-2), sulfonanilide (nimesulide, acts in the thermoregulatory center in the CNS), coxib (etoricoxib and celecoxib, highly selective to COX-2), and NSAIDs without inflammatory activity (acetaminophen and dipyrone), among others [22].

3.1.3 Adverse effects of NSAIDs and recommendations

It is important to be careful with the drug interactions, because they are responsible of multiple effects. It is not recommended to mix NSAIDs with any of these drugs: lithium (increases its toxicity), anticoagulants and/or alcohol (increases risk of GI bleeding), other NSAIDs (increase toxicity and produce kidney failure in the long-term), antihypertensive (Loop) and/or hypoglycemic drugs (decreases hypoglycemic effect), antihypertensive (Loop) and anticonvulsants drugs (increases toxicity of anticonvulsant), antihypertensive drugs such as diuretics or ACE inhibitors (decreases the effect of these drugs), and acetaminophen and alcohol (risk of hepatic damage in patients with previous hepatic damage) [24].

At the level of the gastrointestinal (GI) tract, NSAIDs can cause abdominal pain, nausea, vomit, hemorrhage, gastroduodenal ulcer; also, they can cause peripheral edema and hypertension (particularly if they are nonselective). In the long term, they are associated with congestive heart failure with risk of infarction, hepatic insufficiency, and kidney failure, so they are not recommended for prolonged periods [22, 24, 25].

Furthermore, NSAIDs have demonstrated hypersensitivity in a lot of patients, showing multiple clinical expressions such as pruritus, urticaria, bronchospasm, and anaphylaxis in patients with analgesic intolerance to this group of drugs [26].

Because of all the evidence previously mentioned, the use of selective to COX-2 NSAIDs is associated with less GI adverse effects, therefore these drugs result useful to prevent GI bleeding. However, it is suggested to use a proton bomb inhibitor (PBI) regardless of the NSAID, because to see anti-inflammatory effect, the treatment with NSAIDs must be of 2 weeks [23, 27].

In patients with GI bleeding risk, the use of Celecoxib 200 mg twice a day is recommended, for its low adverse effects, only when there are no cardiovascular risk factors, because of the cardiovascular toxicity of the highly selective to COX-2 NSAIDs [28].

In the group of nonselective NSAIDs, both naproxen and ibuprofen appear to be the safest drugs concerning cardiovascular effects. Moreover, the use of preferential NSAIDs such as meloxicam at a dose of 7.5–15 mg once daily for 2 to 4 weeks achieves pain relief, but it is temporary if the treatment is suspended [28].

Furthermore, Hsieh and cols. in a prospective, randomized, double-blind study of 153 patients with MPS of the trapezius muscle compared the use of topic diclofenac sodium (60 mg) with placebo, 3 times a day for 7 days, concluding it is useful for MPS decreasing the pain without adverse effects [29].

The authors of this chapter suggest individualizing the case, knowing the risks of each patient, and choosing the pharmacologic treatment consciously.

The use of naproxen or ibuprofen with gastric protectors can be fair, and the use of preferential or highly selective to COX-2 NSAIDs without cardiac risk is valid. A pharmacological therapy for 2 weeks could be enough to resolve or improve the clinical condition.

3.1.4 Analgesics

The acetaminophen (Paracetamol) is the most used analgesic; this drug has affinity for the COX-3 at CNS level and almost no affinity for COX-1 and COX-2 [30]. For this reason, an analgesic and antipyretic effect can be achieved, but minimal anti-inflammatory effect. The main advantage is that it acts in a different site from the NSAIDs; this allows enhancing the analgesic effects in addition when it is prescribed with NSAIDs.

Kurita and cols. in a triple-blind study, in 18 patients, compared the effectivity of the diclofenac sodium alone; together with acetaminophen, caffeine, and carisoprodol; and placebo for the treatment of temporomandibular disorders (TMD). They concluded that both diclofenac sodium alone and the group of drugs together reduced the pain until the third day of treatment [31], so acetaminophen in addition with other drugs could be beneficial.

3.1.5 Opioids

These drugs are weak agonists that bind their muscarinic, kappa, and delta receptors at a central level and other tissues getting a similar effect as well as endorphins, altering the pain perception and modulating the painful response of the CNS [32].

These drugs can be combined with other analgesics and NSAIDs staggering the pharmacological therapy in cases of severe pain where it cannot be treated with the previous options. Cigerim and cols. in a double-blind, randomized study of 169 patients with myofascial pain compared naproxen (550 mg) alone, with codeine (30 mg), with dexamethasone (8 mg, single dose), and acetaminophen (550 mg) alone. They concluded that naproxen sodium with codeine has the greatest analgesic effect at the first and fourth week of treatment, suggesting a synergic effect on the part of the codeine unto the naproxen [33]. Moore et al. in a systematic review in 2008 analyzed acetaminophen alone or with codeine (60 mg) for the management of the postoperative pain, showing it can produce pain relief even with a single dose [34].

Although the opioids have shown analgesic effectivity in the chronic musculoskeletal pain, they should be used with care because these drugs can cause abuse, dependence, and adverse effects such as depression of the CNS [35].

For the authors, the use of opioids should be reserved for the last instance in severe pain where multimodal therapy of peripheral action has not solved them.

3.1.6 Musculoskeletal relaxants

The musculoskeletal relaxants act on the CNS interrupting the nociceptive signal but are considered to act in the muscle trigger points [6, 36].

These drugs can be classified into neuromuscular blockers, antispasticity, antispasms, and nerve blockers. The most used are cyclobenzaprine, baclofen, tizanidine, carisoprodol, methocarbamol, and metaxalone, among others [27, 28]. Other type of drugs such as diazepam, Dantrolene and botulinum toxin, can also be mentioned [19].

The most studied musculoskeletal relaxant is cyclobenzaprine, showing analgesic efficacy in MPS with antispasmodic effect in the cervical region; that is why it is recommended as the first treatment option for myogenous TMD. It also has shown better effect with 10 mg than 0.5 mg of clonazepam [6, 23].

Some authors recommend pharmacological treatment with muscle relaxants until 30 days [23, 28]. However, for the authors of this chapter, 2 weeks of musculoskeletal relaxant and multimodal pharmacological therapy are enough to evaluate an improvement of the clinical condition.

The use of ibuprofen with codeine or with cyclobenzaprine has been studied, but has not shown better analgesia and does not even decrease muscle spasms, so it is not recommended as a therapeutic [37, 38].

Also, tizanidine (36 mg daily) has shown pain relief, improvement of sleep, and antispasmodic effect after 5 weeks of treatment for MPS, with doses of 36 mg daily (but lower doses can be used with success) [6].

In addition, Clonazepam (benzodiazepine) as a therapeutic propose acts in the chloride channels increasing the GABA-A receptors; this achieves an inhibition of the pre- and postsynaptic sites on the spinal cord. Even the use of muscle relaxants has therapeutic utility; the depressant effect of CNS can appear [35]. That is why it is important to individualize each therapy and start the treatment with minimal doses and escalate them as required.

3.1.7 Central action pain modulators

In this group are commonly antidepressants, anticonvulsants, and benzodiazepines, among others.

The most common antidepressants are tricyclic antidepressants (TCAs) and serotonin and norepinephrine reuptake inhibitors such as amitriptyline, nortriptyline, duloxetine, and venlafaxine [27].

The gabapentin has shown to be effective for pain relief in myogenous TMD at doses of 300 mg daily, increasing the dose every third day, without exceeding the maximum dose of 4200 mg a day, showing decrease in pain spontaneously at 8 weeks of treatment [27].

Kimos and cols. Evaluated 50 women with chronic masticatory myalgia, comparing the effectivity of gabapentin (300 mg initially) with placebo, concluding that gabapentin was effective for musculoskeletal disorders, suggesting a superiority to the TCAs due to a lower drug interaction [39].

The benzodiazepines have demonstrated good effectiveness for pain. In combined therapy with NSAID, the effect increases. Therefore, benzodiazepines are recommended as a second line and not as initial therapy [27].

Based on this evidence, for the authors, it is convenient to carry out a multimodal treatment for pain management and muscular affection. With the use of drugs with direct effect in the: inflammation, pain, muscle spasm as well as the management of chronic pain at a central level. However, everything depends of the severity of the pain, the individual state of each patient, and the possible pharmacokinetics and pharmacodynamics interactions that may occur. Keep in mind that the MPS affects in its majority the elderly population. For this reason, patients tend to have systemic affections and pharmacologic therapies for those conditions, to consider when to choose a multimodal pharmacological therapy.

4. Physiotherapy

Physiotherapy can be done by the patient at home or by a professional physiotherapist. Myofascial pain can be caused by an excessive functional muscular load, tensional issues (e.g. family problems), bruxism, long dental visit, history of trauma, among others muscles triggers. As a result, we always have to decrease the masticatory function when treating myofascial pain. Physiotherapy carried out in a rehabilitation center or by a physiotherapist for the MPS management is shown in **Table 1** [20].

The physical therapy (or manual) refers to the mobilization of the TMJ, soft tissues of the muscles involved, active and passive movements, gentle isometric tension with resistance, and guided mandibular movements [40].

It is also recommended that a specialist (physiotherapist) performs it, and so do the patient (at home) getting better results [41].

Furthermore, when compared with manual therapy, pain relief is achieved for MPS, followed by dry needling [42].

Extracorporeal shockwave therapy has shown to reduce P substance on the application area and a relief in patients with pain in lower back who undergo this type of therapy [43].

In the case of MPS of the trapezius muscle, it can be treated with extracorporeal shockwave therapy with 6 weekly sessions (1000 pulsations each one). Also, there are reports of similar effects with dry needling, laser, infiltration of trigger points, and so on [43].

Ahi and Sirzai realized a randomized, blind, controlled study in 108 patients with MPS of the neck and upper back; they compared high-intensity laser therapy with dry needling, both together with physical exercise, concluding that both therapies where effective for the MPS management [44].

Regarding to electrode therapy (TENS), Johnson and cols. Conducted a systematic review about the use in patients with any pain condition. TENS showed pain relief during or at the end of each session [45]. Kato and cols. as well in a randomized, controlled study in 18 patients with myogenous TMD compared the use of TENS (with low level pulse of 1.5 sec each one) and laser therapy (of 830–904 nm with power of 100 mW), concluding both therapies can reduce the symptoms of TMD significantly [46].

Physiotherapy at home	Physiotherapy at a rehabilitation center
• Care for TMJ (e.g., maximal mouth opening limitation when eating or yawning, soft diet, superficial warm and moist heat in muscular and articular region, etc.). • Physical (or manual).	• Physical (or manual). • Low laser frequencies. • Extracorporeal shockwave therapy • Transcutaneous Electrical Nerve Stimulation. • Dry needling. • Ozone therapy.

Table 1.
Types of physical therapy for MPS management [3, 20].

Celakil and cols. observed favorable results with ozone therapy for TMD management in a prospective, double-blind, randomized study in 40 patients with chronic masticatory muscle pain. They compared the therapy with bio-oxidative ozone (intensity of 60%) placed on the masticatory muscles and placebo, both 3 times a week for 2 weeks. They concluded that ozone therapy can decrease the pain and improve the mandibular function in myogenous TMD [47].

5. Botulinum toxin

The botulinum toxin (BTX) is produced by the clostridium botulinum bacteria; the action mechanism consists in the inhibition of the acetylcholine on the neuromuscular union, causing muscular paresia. It has also been seen that BTX can act at a CNS level with the central endogenous opioid system, reducing the inflammatory response, being type A the most used for TMD (Botox, Xeomin, and Dysport) [27]. Under this mechanism, the striated muscle is forced to rest of the muscle and masticatory function. Although BTX is widely used for cervical dystonia, overactivity of the bladder, and chronic migraine, there is no consensus for its use for TMD [48].

Systematic reviews about the use of BTX in TMD have been conducted; however, the irregular evidence does not allow to reach a conclusion, even though it has been seen to improve the outcome with conservative treatment [48, 49].

The use of BTX in muscular hypertrophy cases has shown a good response, decreasing the painful symptomatology, getting from high levels of pain (8.2 VAS) to minimal levels (1.8 VAS) after treatment [50].

Some authors recommend the use of 50 IU of BTX initially with 12 week intervals between each infiltration and after a few cycles; BTX can be administered every 6 months reducing the possibility of presenting adverse effects such as facial asymmetry or muscular weakness [51].

For other authors, the application of BTX is indicated only when the patient's condition has not been resolved at all with pharmacologic and physiotherapeutic therapy after 3 weeks of treatment [52].

5.1 BTX application protocol

The first step is to realize an anatomical marking of the zone to identify the affected muscle band and its anatomical relations. These marks are realized exploring the muscle contraction at opening, closing, and maximum intercuspation [53].

The second step is the dilution of the BTX as the supplier recommends [54]. Some suppliers feature diluted BTX, and others need to be diluted in injectable water. The marking of the syringe at the units per ml of solution allows us to quantify the amount of BTX that is going to be injected to each muscle group.

The third step is to perform the asepsis and antisepsis of the area and inject the amount of the desired drug for each muscular condition and for every muscle. For the skin areas, simply perform asepsis with alcohol solution or topical antiseptic. For the intraoral injections, it must be rinsed with chlorhexidine or any other antiseptic solution for oral use (**Figure 5**).

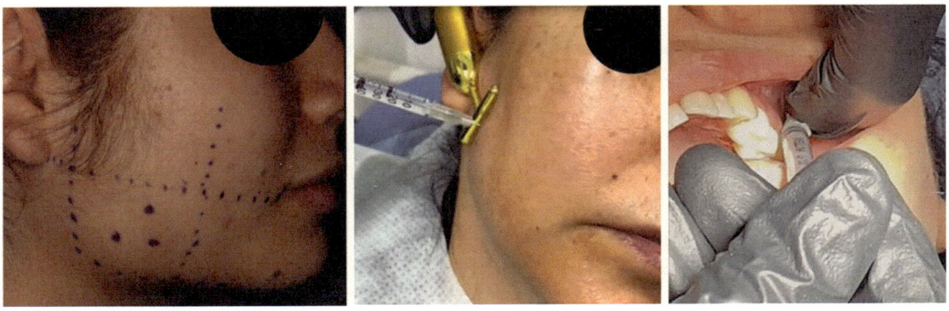

(a) (b) (c)

Figure 5.
A, B. Marks on masseterine region and infiltration of the masseter muscle. C. Intraoral infiltration of lateral pterygoid muscle.

6. Intraoral devices

An occlusal splint is a deprogrammer or a mandibular repositioner to establish the ideal relation between maxilla and mandible, relieving pain and giving correct function. According to the American Academy of Orofacial Pain, the purpose of this device is to give occlusal stability, protect the teeth, redistribute the occlusal forces, relax the muscles, and reduce bruxism [55].

A poorly designed occlusal device or with the wrong material could increase the muscle activity and thus increase the myofascial pain in the patient.

The intraoral devices must meet certain conditions so that the treatment and the orofacial pain control can be effective.

6.1 Basic conditions of efficacy

a. Condylar Stability

b. Guard Design

c. Permanent Action

d. Correct and Timely Adjustments of the Guard

6.2 Condylar stability

The intraoral device must be designed considering the dental contact and the stability at a condylar level. Patients with myofascial pain frequently have an important level of temporomandibular dysfunction and dental alterations. All these situations can cause the patient to present a "double occlusion." This condition refers to a forced occlusion where the patient feels more comfortable but can be prejudicial for the joint and other anatomical structures [56].

A correct design of the intraoral device will provide the patient the necessary occlusal stability to not having to look for a new mandibular position, so we will eliminate that "double" occlusion [57].

6.3 Guard ydesign

The elaboration of the intraoral device requires an articulator mounting. Through the facial arch, we will determine the position of the maxillary occlusal plane and thus find the appropriate maxilla–mandible relation for the patient. A registration must be made with interoclusal wax without teeth contact, to ensure the elimination of the proprioception with the selected technique by the operator seeking to establish the condyles in the most stable possible position [58].

The diagnostic mounting allows realizing a detailed analysis of the occlusion, determining the existence of any fulcrum that could cause any sort of pry over the TMJ, as well as interferences on the mandibular excursion. This same diagnostic mounting could be used for the design of the intraoral device; we could determine the thickness of it by separating the first point of contact by 2–3 mm; after that, we will try to simulate with the splint a perfect functional occlusion giving what is known as "mutually protected occlusion." This can be achieved by having uniform contacts and with the same intensity in every work cusp of the opposite arch and a slight disocclusion of a thousandth of an inch in the anterior teeth. The anterior ramp of the intraoral device should have an inclination of 45° approximately, which gives immediate posterior disocclusion in any mandibular movement (laterality and protrusion) [58].

The treatment with splint should be considered as a permanent action in order to get the desired results; that is why patient cooperation is indispensable. The splint should stay in the mouth 24 hours a day, 7 days of the week, so patients should perform all their activities with the splint. The splint can only be retired after each meal in order to perform the dental and guard hygiene [59].

6.4 Correct and timely adjustments of the guard

The treatment with the splint must have follow-up for several months, at least 3 to 4 months, in which the splint will be checked, verifying the permanence of the ideal simultaneous dental contacts and with the same intensity. At the beginning, those revisions should be done every week, posteriorly fortnightly; however, when we will get stability, they could be monthly [58]. If the adjustments are not performed, which consists in the wear of possible interferences or premature points in the acrylic, the patient could experience periods of incommodity or even an increase of the pain. That is why adequate adjustments are important.

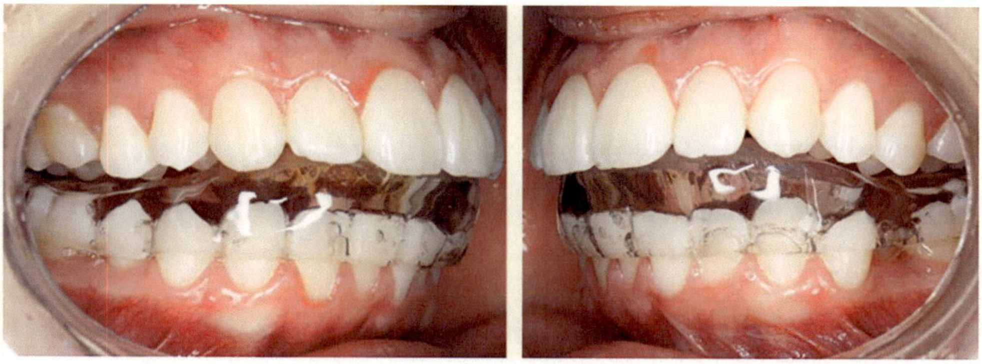

Figure 6.
A, B. Lower gnathologic guard.

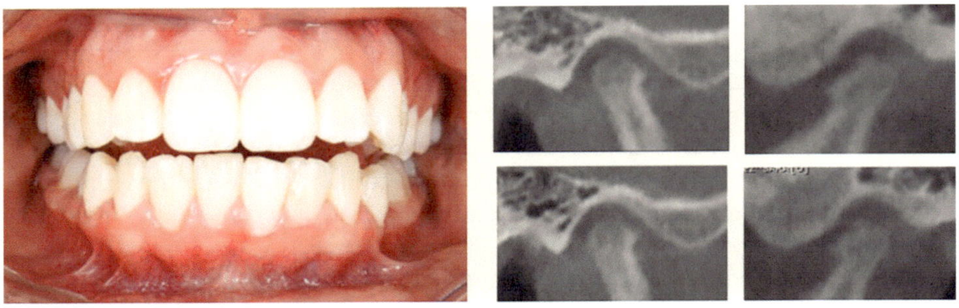

(a) (b)

Figure 7.
A. Posttreatment occlusion. B–E. TC scan after 8 months of treatment. Note the corticalization of the condylar processes and the real malocclusion ready to be treated with surgical-orthodontic treatment.

6.5 Clinical case

We present a case of a female patient of 15 years old, who presents bilateral clicking and pain on the masseter muscle, in the left ear, neck, upper back, and shoulders. We carry out: CT scan of both mandibular condyles (with signs of active degenerative process), diagnostic mounting of casts (it was observed the change of occlusion from Class I to Class II with a considerably increased projection) (**Figure 4**).

The gnathologic guard is done with multiple contacts and with anterior guide (**Figure 6**). Achieving favorable outcome as all the symptoms disappear after 2 months of treatment without needing of other alternative therapies (e.g., pharmacologic). The tomography showed that the degenerative process stopped and achieved recorticalization of the condyles and articular eminence (**Figure 7**).

Author details

Leandro Díez-Suárez[1*], Rodrigo Garay Symor[2] and Arturo Ivan Espinosa Carlos[3]

1 National Autonomous University of Mexico UNAM, Mexico City, Mexico

2 National Autonomous University of Mexico UNAM, Mexico State, Mexico

3 Advanced Education in Orthodontics, Mexico City, Mexico

*Address all correspondence to: ledisuar@gmail.com

References

[1] Alomar X, Medrano J, Cabratosa J, Clavero JA, Lorente M, Serra I, et al. Anatomy of the temporomandibular joint. Seminars in Ultrasound, CT, and MR. 2007;**28**(3):170-183

[2] Liu F, Steinkeler A. Epidemiology, diagnosis, and treatment of temporomandibular disorders. Dental Clinics of North America. 2013;**57**(3):465-479

[3] Tanaka E, Detamore MS, Mercuri LG. Degenerative disorders of the temporomandibular joint: Etiology, diagnosis, and treatment. Journal of Dental Research. 2008;**87**(4):296-307

[4] Hisatomi M, Munhoz L, Asaumi J, Arita ES. Parotid mandibular bone defect: A case report emphasizing imaging features in plain radiographs and magnetic resonance imaging. Imaging Science in Dentistry. 2017;**47**(4):269-273

[5] Ohrbach R, Slade GD, Bair E, Rathnayaka N, Diatchenko L, Greenspan JD, et al. Premorbid and concurrent predictors of TMD onset and persistence. European Journal of Pain. 2020;**24**(1):145-158

[6] Borg-Stein J, Iaccarino MA. Myofascial pain syndrome treatments. Physical Medicine and Rehabilitation Clinics of North America. 2014;**25**(2):357-374

[7] Tran C, Ghahreman K, Huppa C, Gallagher JE. Management of temporomandibular disorders: A rapid review of systematic reviews and guidelines. International Journal of Oral and Maxillofacial Surgery. 2022;**51**(9):1211-1225

[8] Lomas J, Gurgenci T, Jackson C, Campbell D. Temporomandibular dysfunction. Australian Journal of General Practice. 2018;**47**(4):212-215

[9] Chan NHY, Ip CK, Li DTS, Leung YY. Diagnosis and treatment of Myogenous temporomandibular disorders: A clinical update. Diagnostics (Basel). 2022;**12**(12):2914

[10] Nascimento MM, Vasconcelos BC, Porto GG, Ferdinanda G, Nogueira CM, Raimundo RD. Physical therapy and anesthetic blockage for treating temporomandibular disorders: A clinical trial. Medicina Oral, Patología Oral y Cirugía Bucal. 2013;**18**(1):e81-e85

[11] Donlon WC, Truta MP, Eversole LR. A modified auriculotemporal nerve block for regional anesthesia of the temporomandibular joint. Journal of Oral and Maxillofacial Surgery. 1984;**42**(8):544-545

[12] Mejersjö C, Pauli N. Ear symptoms in patients with orofacial pain and dysfunction—An explorative study on different TMD symptoms, occlusion and habits. Cllinical and Experimental Dental Research. 2021;7(6):1167-1174

[13] Vlăduțu D, Popescu SM, Mercuț R, Ionescu M, Scrieciu M, Glodeanu AD, et al. Associations between bruxism, stress, and manifestations of temporomandibular disorder in young students. International Journal of Environmental Research and Public Health. 2022;**19**(9):5415

[14] Fernandes G, Franco AL, Siqueira JT, Gonçalves DA, Camparis CM. Sleep bruxism increases the risk for painful temporomandibular disorder, depression and non-specific physical symptoms. Journal of Oral Rehabilitation. 2012;**39**(7):538-544

[15] Dhanrajani PJ, Jonaidel O. Trismus: Aetiology, differential diagnosis and treatment. Dental Update. 2002;**29**(2):88-94

[16] Taşkaya-Yilmaz N, Oğütcen-Toller M. Magnetic resonance imaging evaluation of temporomandibular joint disc deformities in relation to type of disc displacement. Journal of Oral and Maxillofacial Surgery. 2001;**59**(8):860-865 discussion 865-866

[17] Fushima K, Inui M, Sato S. Dental asymmetry in temporomandibular disorders. Journal of Oral Rehabilitation. 1999;**26**(9):752-756

[18] Ivan Urits I, Charipova K, Gress K, Schaaf AL, Gupta S, Kiernan HC, et al. Treatment and management of myofascial pain syndrome. Best Practice & Research Clinical Anaesthesiology. 2020;**34**(3):427-448

[19] Heir GM. The efficacy of pharmacologic treatment of temporomandibular disorders. Oral and Maxillofacial Surgery Clinics of North America. 2018;**30**(3):279-285

[20] Ferrillo M, Giudice A, Marotta N, Fortunato F, Di Venere D, Ammendolia A, et al. Pain management and rehabilitation for central sensitization in temporomandibular disorders: A comprehensive review. International Journal of Molecular Sciences. 2022;**23**(20):12164

[21] García-Rayado G, Navarro M, Lanas A. NSAID induced gastrointestinal damage and designing GI-sparing NSAIDs. Expert Review of Clinical Pharmacology. 2018;**11**(10):1031-1043

[22] Bacchi S, Palumbo P, Sponta A, Coppolino MF. Clinical pharmacology of non-steroidal anti-inflammatory drugs: A review. Anti-Inflammatory & Anti-Allergy Agents in Medicinal Chemistry. 2012;**11**(1):52-64

[23] Hersh EV, Balasubramaniam R, Pinto A. Pharmacologic management of temporomandibular disorders. Oral and Maxillofacial Surgery Clinics of North America. 2008;**20**(2):197-210

[24] Hersh EV, Pinto A, Moore PA. Adverse drug interactions involving common prescription and over-the-counter analgesic agents. Clinical Therapeutics. 2007;**29**(Suppl):2477-2497

[25] Grosser T, Smith EM, FitzGerald GA. Pharmacotherapy of inflammation, fever, pain, and gout. In: Brunton LL, Hilal R, Knollmann BC, editors. Goodman & Gilman's: The Pharmacological Basis of Therapeutics. 13th ed. USA: McGraw Hill Education; 2019. pp. 673-684

[26] Celik G, Erkekol FO, Bavbek S, Dursun B, Misirligil Z. Long-term use and tolerability of cyclooxygenase-2 inhibitors in patients with analgesic intolerance. Annals of Allergy, Asthma & Immunology. 2005;**95**(1):33-37

[27] Andre A, Kang J, Dym H. Pharmacologic treatment for temporomandibular and temporomandibular joint disorders. Oral and Maxillofacial Surgery Clinics of North America. 2022;**34**(1):49-59

[28] Ouanounou A, Goldberg M, Haas DA. Pharmacotherapy in temporomandibular disorders: A review. Journal of the Canadian Dental Association. 2017;**83**:h7

[29] Hsieh LF, Hong CZ, Chern SH, Chen CC. Efficacy and side effects of diclofenac patch in treatment of patients with myofascial pain syndrome of the upper trapezius. Journal of Pain and Symptom Management. 2010;**39**(1):116-125

[30] Botting R, Ayoub SS. COX-3 and the mechanism of action of paracetamol/acetaminophen. Prostaglandins, Leukotrienes, and Essential Fatty Acids. 2005;**72**(2):85-87

[31] Kurita Varoli F, Sucena Pita M, Sato S, Issa JP, do Nascimento C, Pedrazzi V. Analgesia evaluation of 2 NSAID drugs as adjuvant in management of chronic temporomandibular disorders. Scientific World Journal. 2015;**2015**:359152

[32] Inturrisi CE. Clinical pharmacology of opioids for pain. The Clinical Journal of Pain. 2002;**18**(4 Suppl):S3-S13

[33] Cigerim L, Kaplan V. Analgesic efficacy of naproxen-codeine, naproxen+dexamethasone, and naproxen on myofascial pain: A randomized double-blind controlled trial. Cranio. 2023;**41**(2):119-125

[34] Moore A, Collins S, Carroll D, McQuay H, Edwards J. Single dose paracetamol (acetaminophen), with and without codeine, for postoperative pain. Cochrane Database of Systematic Review. 2000;(4). Article ID: CD001547. DOI: 10.1002/14651858.CD001547

[35] Galasso A, Urits I, An D, Nguyen D, Borchart M, Yazdi C, et al. A comprehensive review of the treatment and management of myofascial pain syndrome. Current Pain and Headache Reports. 2020;**24**(8):43

[36] Desai MJ, Bean MC, Heckman TW, Jayaseelan D, Moats N, Nava A. Treatment of myofascial pain. Pain Management. 2013;**3**(1):67-79

[37] Turturro MA, Frater CR, D'Amico FJ. Cyclobenzaprine with ibuprofen versus ibuprofen alone in acute myofascial strain: A randomized, double-blind clinical trial. Annals of Emergency Medicine. 2003;**41**(6):818-826

[38] Childers MK, Borenstein D, Brown RL, Gershon S, Hale ME, Petri M, et al. Low-dose cyclobenzaprine versus combination therapy with ibuprofen for acute neck or back pain with muscle spasm: A randomized trial. Current Medical Research and Opinion. 2005;**21**(9):1485-1493

[39] Kimos P, Biggs C, Mah J, Heo G, Rashiq S, Thie NM, et al. Analgesic action of gabapentin on chronic pain in the masticatory muscles: A randomized controlled trial. Pain. 2007;**127**(1-2):151-160

[40] de Melo LA, Bezerra de Medeiros AK, Campos MFTP, Machado B, de Resende CM, Barbosa GAS, et al. Manual therapy in the treatment of myofascial pain related to temporomandibular disorders: A systematic review. Journal of Oral & Facial Pain and Headache. 2020;**34**(2):141-148

[41] Tuncer AB, Ergun N, Tuncer AH, Karahan S. Effectiveness of manual therapy and home physical therapy in patients with temporomandibular disorders: A randomized controlled trial. Journal of Bodywork and Movement Therapies. 2013;**17**(3):302-308

[42] Menéndez-Torre Á, Pintado-Zugasti AM, Zaldivar JNC, García-Bermejo P, Gómez-Costa D, Molina-Álvarez M, et al. Effectiveness of deep dry needling versus manual therapy in the treatment of myofascial temporomandibular disorders: A systematic review and network meta-analysis. Chiropractic & Manual Therapies. 2023;**31**(1):46

[43] De la Corte-Rodríguez H, Román-Belmonte JM, Rodríguez-Damiani BA, Vázquez-Sasot A, Rodríguez-Merchán EC. Extracorporeal shock wave therapy for the treatment of musculoskeletal pain: A narrative review. Healthcare (Basel). 2023;**11**(21):2830

[44] Ahi ED, Sirzai H. Comparison of the effectiveness of dry needling and high-intensity laser therapy in the treatment of myofascial pain syndrome: A randomized single-blind controlled study. Lasers in Medical Science. 2022;**38**(1):3

[45] Johnson MI, Paley CA, Jones G, Mulvey MR, Wittkopf PG. Efficacy and safety of transcutaneous electrical nerve stimulation (TENS) for acute and chronic pain in adults: A systematic review and meta-analysis of 381 studies (the meta-TENS study). BMJ Open. 2022;**12**(2):e051073

[46] Kato MT, Kogawa EM, Santos CN, Conti PC. TENS and low-level laser therapy in the management of temporomandibular disorders. Journal of Applied Oral Science. 2006;**14**(2):130-135

[47] Celakil T, Muric A, Gokcen Roehlig B, Evlioglu G, Keskin H. Effect of high-frequency bio-oxidative ozone therapy for masticatory muscle pain: A double-blind randomised clinical trial. Journal of Oral Rehabilitation. 2017;**44**(6):442-451

[48] Thambar S, Kulkarni S, Armstrong S, Nikolarakos D. Botulinum toxin in the management of temporomandibular disorders: A systematic review. The British Journal of Oral & Maxillofacial Surgery. 2020;**58**(5):508-519

[49] Gil-Martínez A, Paris-Alemany A, López-de-Uralde-Villanueva I, La Touche R. Management of pain in patients with temporomandibular disorder (TMD): Challenges and solutions. Journal of Pain Research. 2018;**11**:571-587

[50] Farrier JN, Farrier S, Haworth S, Beech AN. Can we justify the continued use of botulinum toxin A in the management of myofascial pain? The British Journal of Oral & Maxillofacial Surgery. 2020;**58**(9):1133-1138

[51] González MF, Miranda LM, Malagón HH, González AV. Use of botulinum toxin for treatment of hypertrophy of the masseter muscle. Cirugía Plástica Ibero-Latinoamericana. 2012;**38**(3):297-302

[52] Yoshida K. Effects of botulinum toxin type a on pain among trigeminal neuralgia, myofascial temporomandibular disorders, and oromandibular dystonia. Toxins. 2021;**13**:605

[53] Serrera-Figallo MA, Ruiz-de-León-Hernández G, Torres-Lagares D, Castro-Araya A, Torres-Ferrerosa O, Hernández-Pacheco E, et al. Use of botulinum toxin in orofacial clinical practice. Toxins (Basel). 2020;**12**(2):112

[54] Kandhari R, Kaur I, Gupta J, Al-Niaimi F. Microdroplet botulinum toxin: A review. Journal of Cutaneous and Aesthetic Surgery. 2022;**15**(2):101-107

[55] Albagieh H, Alomran I, Binakresh A, Alhatarisha N, Almeteb M, Khalaf Y, et al. Occlusal splints-types and effectiveness in temporomandibular disorder management. The Saudi Dental Journal. 2023;**35**(1):70-79

[56] Ahmed MMS, Shi D, Al-Somairi MAA, Alhashimi N, Almashraqi AA, Musa M, et al. Three dimensional evaluation of the skeletal and temporomandibular joint changes following stabilization splint therapy in patients with temporomandibular joint disorders and mandibular deviation: A retrospective study. BMC Oral Health. 2023;**23**(1):18

[57] Al-Moraissi EA, Farea R, Qasem KA, Al-Wadeai MS, Al-Sabahi ME, Al-Iryani GM. Effectiveness of occlusal

splint therapy in the management of temporomandibular disorders: Network meta-analysis of randomized controlled trials. International Journal of Oral and Maxillofacial Surgery. 2020;**49**(8):1042-1056

[58] Lundeen TF. Occlusal splint fabrication. The Journal of Prosthetic Dentistry. 1979;**42**(5):588-591

[59] Matsumoto H, Tsukiyama Y, Kuwatsuru R, Koyano K. The effect of intermittent use of occlusal splint devices on sleep bruxism: A 4-week observation with a portable electromyographic recording device. Journal of Oral Rehabilitation. 2015;**42**(4):251-258

Chapter 3

Current Concepts in Minimal-Invasive Surgical Approach of Temporomandibular Joint Disorders

Mario Santagata, Ciro Emiliano Boschetti, Giuseppe Colella, Carmelo Consiglio, Roberta Magliulo, Roberta Sivo, Davide Morlando, Annalisa Pollice, David Guida, Ivo Ferrieri, Salvatore D'Amato, Luigi Rugge, Gianpaolo Tartaro and Fabrizio Chirico

Abstract

Nowadays temporomandibular disorders (TMD) management has changed dramatically as more advanced knowledge regarding physiopathology has developed and treatment strategies have evolved into less invasive and multidisciplinary as TMD multifactorial nature. According to our cranio maxillofacial experience, the purpose of this chapter is to present a comprehensive overview of TMD minimally invasive surgical approach to achieve outcomes in a reasonably conservative and cost-effective manner, based on the massive amount of ongoing research in the most recent literature. The chapter is divided into five main sections. The first consists of an overview of temporomandibular disorders preoperative assessment. The second is a description of operative strategies decision-making presenting indications for individual rational treatments. The third presents a description of operative techniques current view as arthrocentesis and injections of hyaluronic acid and blood-derived stem cells. The fourth describes what we evaluate and the role of arthrocentesis in various temporomandibular disorders. The fifth section underlines future surgical prospects with advancements in technology and regenerative medicine, meeting the criteria of translational TMD management.

Keywords: temporomandibular disorder, temporomandibular joint, facial pain, conservative treatment, minimally invasive procedure, arthrocentesis

1. Introduction

1.1 Temporomandibular disorders clinical features in multidisciplinary treatment approach

Temporomandibular disorders (TMD) [1–10] constitute a broad category encompassing various musculoskeletal conditions characterized by pain and/or dysfunction in the masticatory muscles, temporomandibular joints (TMJ), and related structures (**Figure 1**).

It stands out as the most prevalent form of non-odontogenic orofacial pain, presenting symptoms such as facial/head pain, TMJ discomfort (**Figure 2**), tooth-related pain, restricted jaw movement, and audible sounds in the TMJ during jaw activities. Despite its primary definition rooted in orofacial pain and dysfunction, TMD often coexists with other ailments, including headaches, fibromyalgia, irritable bowel syndrome, tinnitus, chronic fatigue syndrome, depression, and sleep disturbances. Ongoing research emphasizes the intricate biopsychosocial aspects of common

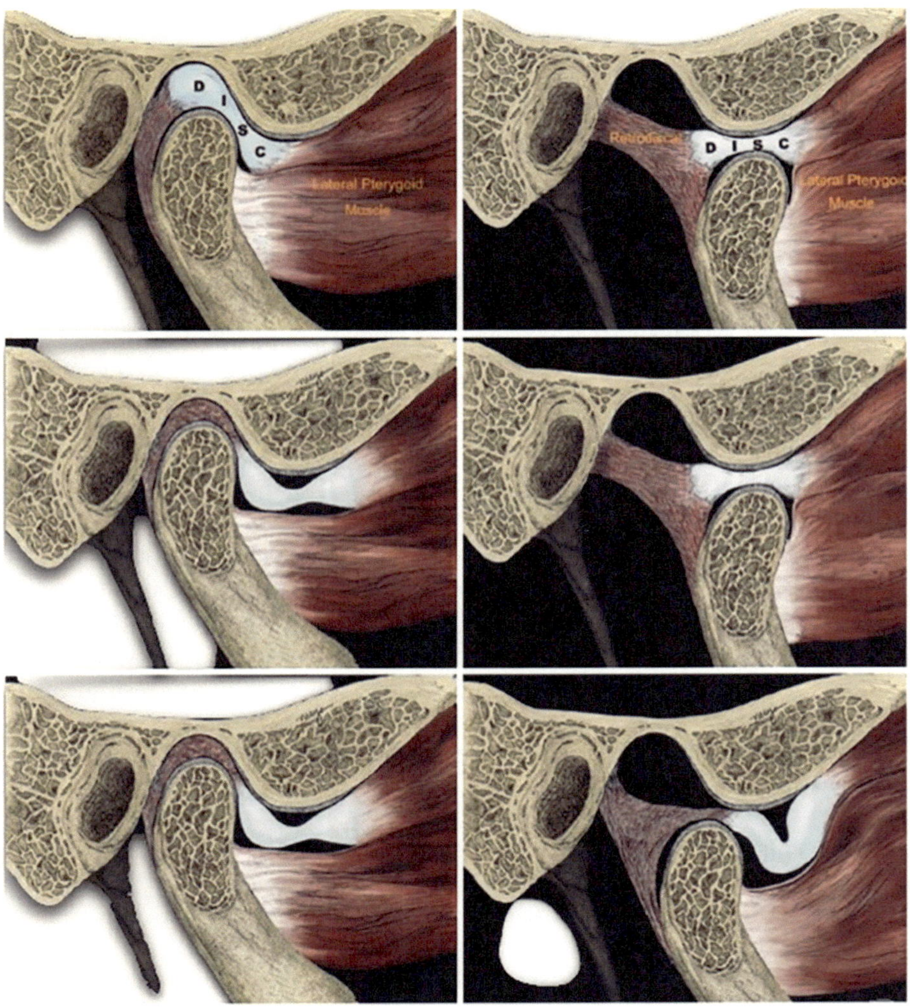

Figure 1.
Sequence of internal derangement in temporomandibular disorders.

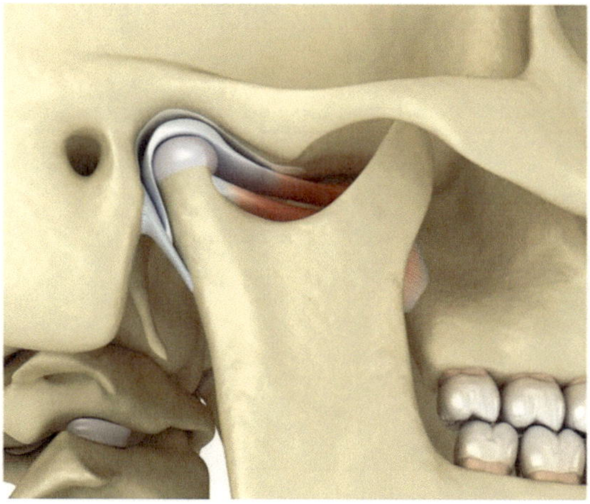

Figure 2.
TMJ anatomical illustration.

painful TMD (myalgia and/or arthralgia) and their interconnectedness with overall health, reinforcing the understanding of TMD as a complex and multifaceted condition. Thus, appropriate treatment should accomplish a multidisciplinary team in the diagnosis of surgical, operative, functional, and/or pharmacological approaches.

Implementing care pathways geared toward facilitating early diagnosis and effective management holds the potential to enhance prognosis, elevate quality of life, and curtail healthcare costs for TMD patients. Proactive measures in diagnosis and minimally invasive surgical intervention can play a pivotal role in mitigating the impact of TMD, offering a more favorable outlook for individuals navigating this challenging condition.

1.2 Temporomandibular disorders preoperative diagnosis

Over time, various forms of temporomandibular disorders (TMD) assessment have been proposed, with the Diagnostic Criteria for temporomandibular disorders (DC/TMD) being among the most widely used as an evidence-based set of tools for diagnosing TMD [11–16]. The DC/TMD provides a standardized and operationalized approach to physically examine the masticatory structures described in axis I (**Table 1**) while also incorporating a screening process for psychosocial and comorbid factors in axis II (**Table 2**) [6].

Moreover, DC/TMD classification introduces a validated temporomandibular disorders (TMD) pain screener designed to identify pain-related disturbances in any clinical setting (**Table 3**). If a patient screens positively using the TMD pain screener, it suggests the need for further, more in-depth evaluation for potential TMD-related issues. This expanded approach aimed to provide a more thorough and nuanced understanding of the psychosocial aspects associated with TMD conditions in order to plan the most appropriate therapeutic approach.

1.3 Prognosis of temporomandibular disorders and timing of surgical approach

Upon re-examination of adults diagnosed with incident temporomandibular disorders (TMD) approximately 8 months after the initial diagnosis, a noteworthy

1. Muscle: • Myofascial suffering. • Myofascial suffering plus limitation in mouth opening.
2. Disk displacement: • Disk displacement with reduction. • Disk displacement without reduction, with limited opening. • Disk displacement without reduction, without limited opening.
3. Arthralgia, arthritis, arthrosis: • Arthralgia • Osteoarthritis. • Osteoarthrosis.

Table 1.
DC/TMD axis I.

Most common pain-related temporomandibular disorders. 1. Myalgia: • Local myalgia. • Myofascial pain. • Myofascial pain with referral. 2. Arthralgia 3. Headache attributed to TMD
Intra-Articular TMD. 1. Disk displacement with reduction. 2. Disk displacement with reduction, with intermittent locking. 3. Disk displacement without reduction, with limited opening. 4. Disk displacement without reduction, without limited opening. 5. Degenerative TMJ disease. 6. Subluxation.

Table 2.
DC/TMD axis II.

observation was made: 51% of these individuals no longer met the criteria for TMD. This suggests a substantial rate of remission or resolution within a relatively short timeframe following the initial diagnosis [8]. After 5 years, remittance rates were reported to be 49%, indicating a considerable proportion of individuals experiencing relief from TMD symptoms without any treatment [9]. These findings highlight the importance of considering the temporal aspect and potential fluctuations in TMD symptoms when evaluating the prognosis of individuals diagnosed with this condition, according to scheduling the timing of the surgical approach. Moreover, these clinical elements demonstrate the complex relationship between clinical presentation and structural diagnoses in the temporomandibular joint, suggesting that the presence of certain intra-articular conditions may not necessarily align with the patient's reported symptoms or functional treatment outcomes over time.

1. In 1 month, how long did TMJ's suffering last? i. No suffering (0). ii. Intermittent suffering (1). iii. Constant suffering (2).
2. In 1 month, did you have TMJ suffering on awaking? i. No (0). ii. Yes (1).
3. In 1 month, did those actions modify your TMJ suffering? a. Biting hard food: i. No (0). ii. Yes (1). b. Mouth opening or jaw movements: i. No (0). ii. Yes (1). c. Jaws habit: to clench, grind, chew: i. No (0). ii. Yes (1). d. Other jaws movements: i. No (0). ii. Yes (1).

Table 3.
TMD pain screener.

1.4 Focus on temporomandibular disorders-related pain in preoperative patient assessment

Painful temporomandibular disorders (TMD) are recognized as biopsychosocial and multifactorial conditions, making it highly unlikely to pinpoint a singular cause in any given patient. The etiology of painful TMD is hypothesized to involve two key domains: the individual's psychological profile and a state of pain amplification. The development of painful temporomandibular disorders (TMD) and associated comorbid symptoms (irritable bowel syndrome, insomnia) and nonspecific orofacial symptoms (stiffness, fatigue) involves a complex interplay of biological, psychological, and social vulnerabilities interacting with contextual and environmental stressors. This intricate web of factors can lead to the manifestation of TMD, whether or not there are identifiable initiating events such as macro trauma (**Figure 3**), micro trauma (**Figure 4**) and/or anatomic factors (**Figure 5**).

The degree to which these factors contribute can either perpetuate symptoms or contribute to the recovery process even if the most appropriate approach is chosen. This holistic perspective acknowledges the dynamic and multifaceted nature of painful TMD, emphasizing the need for a comprehensive approach that considers those aspects in understanding and managing this condition. Although the exact pathophysiology of painful temporomandibular disorders (TMD) is not fully understood, various interconnected factors have been suggested to explain how genetic, emotional, pain perception and social influences combine to

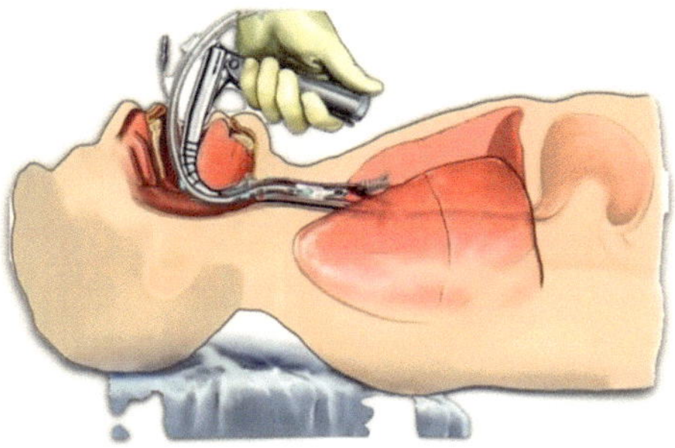

Figure 3.
Oro-tracheal intubation as example of microtrauma.

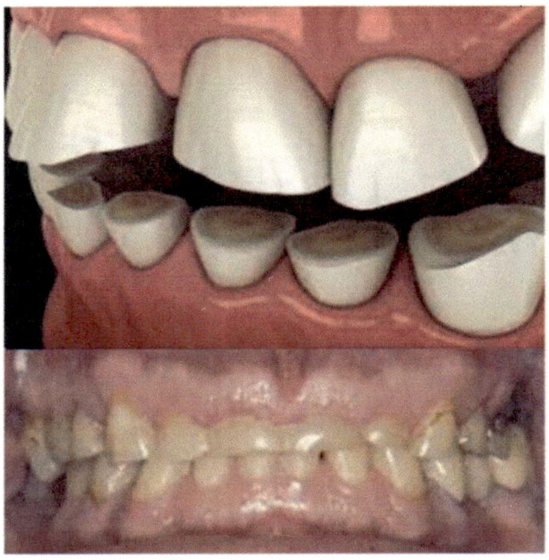

Figure 4.
Dento-skeletal malocclusion as example of microtrauma.

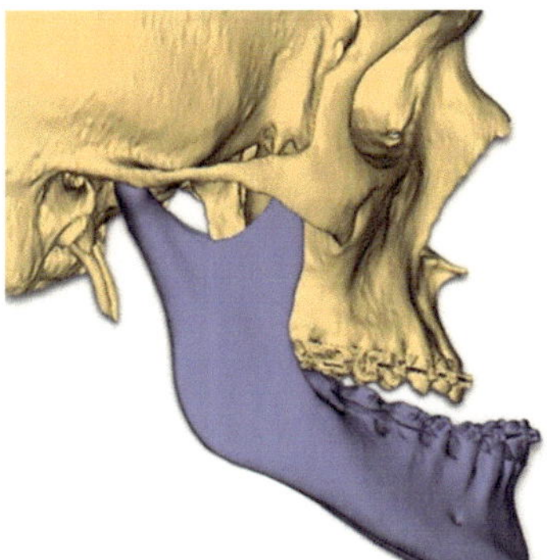

Figure 5.
Cranio maxillofacial deformity and malocclusion as anatomic factors leading to temporomandibular disorders.

influence individuals to maintain or trigger pain associated with TMD. Research focused on chronic suffering and TMJ disorders has identified possible neurological, hormonal, and inflammation-related pathways involved in these conditions.

The presence of inflammation may have a more pronounced role in temporomandibular joint (TMJ) arthralgia and degenerative joint disease (DJD), as evidenced by associations with altered markers in the joints or synovial fluid. This evidence is the core of the current and future perspective of a minimally invasive approach with the aim to both decrease the intracapsular inflammation and contextually regenerate the damaged tissue.

2. Management of temporomandibular disorders

Because of the complex biological and psychological etiological factors of temporomandibular disorders (TMD), treatment strategies that focus only on locoregional anatomic aspects, such as jaw positioning, are inconsistent with the modern evidence in this pathology. Otherwise, effective management could emphasize treating the overall pain involvement, enhancing mandibular function, and taking psychological elements into account. Temporomandibular Joint (TMJ) noises and intra-articular conditions, such as disc displacement (DD) or Degenerative Joint Disease (DJD), should guide treatment options only when they are linked to pain or significant functional limitations, like difficulty fully opening the mouth because of locking [16]. It is highly recommended to provide instruction about the benignity of TMD and to offer a clear, albeit provisional, diagnosis at the first patient assessment. This strategy seeks to reduce the unnecessary distress often caused by doubts related to clinical symptomatology. Furthermore, reversible or conservative approaches, supported by international consensus through thorough evaluation of risks and benefits, are advised as the primary course of treatment. A significant percentage of incident TMD cases exhibit a self-limiting course, progressing to remission within the initial 6–15 months [17]. Treatment plans may incorporate multimodal strategies tailored to case complexity and the contributing factors identified for each patient. This individualized approach acknowledges the diverse and multifaceted nature of TMD, promoting effective and patient-centered management.

2.1 Reversible and conservative treatments

Self-care techniques: A self-management program for temporomandibular disorders (TMD) can encompass several essential elements. These may include identifying, examining, and avoiding oral habits such as nail biting or gum chewing. It also involves guidance on sleep hygiene, recommendations for reducing caffeine intake, adopting a diet that minimizes pain, practicing massage, engaging in relaxing exercises, applying thermal bathing, and using calming practices like diaphragmatic breath. Currently, there is a lack of data to ascertain what TMD diagnoses require adjustments to the self-management approach [18]. Beyond the initial management phase, these self-care strategies are vital, enabling patients to exercise a degree of patient independence in managing symptomology during recurrent TMJ disorders spots or recurrence.

Intraoral devices: Numerous reviews have investigated the effects of occlusal devices on pain associated with Temporomandibular Disorder (TMD). These reviews indicate that stabilization splints—whether made of hard acrylic or soft polyethylene, which fully cover the occlusal surface (**Figure 6**)—tend to provide short-term relief when worn nightly on the upper or lower jaw, particularly in comparison to the absence of treatment. However, the evidence remains

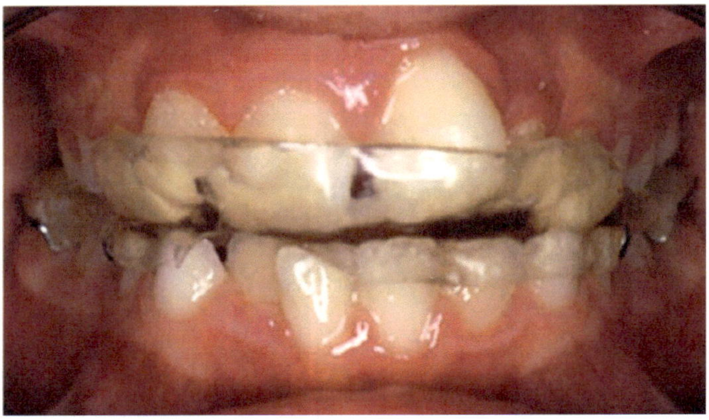

Figure 6.
Stabilization splints as treatment of temporomandibular disorder (TMD) pain.

inconclusive when these appliances are compared to placebo treatments, such as non-occluding palatal splints. Additionally, stabilization splints demonstrate similar effectiveness in alleviating TMD pain when compared to interventions such as physical therapy, behavioral medicine, and acupuncture. It is worth noting that partial coverage appliances like nociceptive trigeminal inhibition and over-the-counter mouthguards may be associated with adverse complications, including unintended occlusal changes [19].

A review and meta-analysis [20] provided valuable insights into the pharmacotherapeutic and therapeutic interventions for managing chronic orofacial pain, particularly in the context of Temporomandibular Disorder (TMD):

2.1.1 Pharmacotherapy

1. Muscle relaxants: Cyclobenzaprine has been supported as effective for short-term relief (approximately 3 weeks) of TMD muscular pain. This highlights its role in acute management strategies.

2. Topical treatments: The review points to preliminary evidence for topical ointment and melatonin's potential effect in reducing TMD muscle pain, although these findings are based on limited studies.

3. NSAIDs: There is consistent evidence supporting the efficacy of nonsteroidal anti-inflammatories in alleviating chronic TMD joint pain, making them a staple option in TMD management [20].

4. Off-label prescription of neuromodulators: The use of various off-label medications, including tricyclic antidepressants, serotonin-noradrenaline reuptake inhibitors, benzodiazepine, gabapentin and pregabalin, is noted, especially in more complex pain scenarios involving central sensitization and comorbid conditions. The acknowledgment of their predominant evidence from other chronic pain conditions calls for cautious application in TMD treatment.

5. Comorbidities: The selection of pharmacotherapy should also consider comorbid conditions (e.g., headaches, sleep disturbances, anxiety [21]), highlighting the

need for a comprehensive assessment of the patient's medical history to avoid medication interactions or complications.

2.1.2 Psychological and multimodal therapies

a. Cognitive-behavioral therapy (CBT): In the literature, reviews indicate that CBT yields significant long-term benefits for TMD pain, depression, and functional interference. The combination of CBT with biofeedback offers additional benefits, particularly for patients with pronounced psychological symptoms.

b. Biofeedback: While biofeedback was found to be effective in reducing pain, its combination with CBT did not result in significantly greater outcomes than CBT alone [22].

2.1.3 Physical therapy

1. Interventions for muscle pain: Clinical trials have shown that interventions such as jaw mobilization and stretching (**Figure** 7) are effective in improving muscle stiffness and jaw movement compared to standard education and other modalities [23].

2. Joint pain management: Physical therapy approaches that utilize jaw mobilization or stretching demonstrate improvements in outcomes for TMD joint pain.

3. Combinations of exercises: Combining strengthening and coordination exercises with mobilization and postural adjustments has shown positive results, enhancing both joint pain relief and improved mobility compared to control conditions [23].

In summary, the management of TMD is multifaceted, requiring a blend of pharmacotherapeutic measures, psychological interventions, and physical therapy modalities tailored to individual patient profiles. Comprehensive evaluations of patients, considering both physical and psychological health, are essential for optimizing treatment outcomes and addressing the complexities of chronic orofacial pain syndromes.

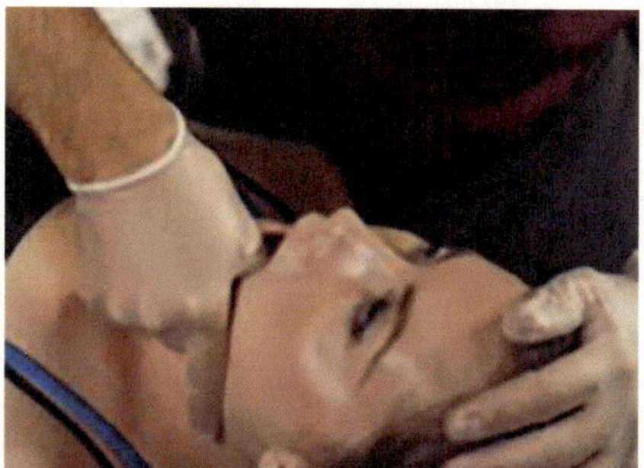

Figure 7.
Postural exercises as physical therapy of temporomandibular disorders.

2.2 Irreversible and invasive treatments

Considering the biological, psychological, and social roots of temporomandibular disorder, along with its typical progression and the effectiveness of reversible and conservative treatments, only a limited number of chronic TMD suffering cases that experience considerable functional limitations may gain advantages from minimally invasive or invasive interventions. At present, there is a lack of adequate tools to forecast TMD outcomes and the effectiveness of various treatments [24]. It is crucial to note that the failure of reversible and conservative treatments alone does not necessarily indicate the need for irreversible and invasive interventions. Moreover, as chronic TMD often involves long-term symptom management for recurrent episodes, it is important to set appropriate expectations for patients.

Surgical management in temporomandibular joint articular disorders (disc substitution or degenerative joint illness) and temporomandibular disorder arthralgia:

A literature review demonstrated similar results of arthrocentesis, arthroscopy, and physical therapy on pain levels, jaw mobility, and functionality in patients with disc displacement (DD) without reduction. An alternative review also reported comparable outcomes for arthrocentesis, arthroscopy, and discectomy (see **Figures 8** and **9**). Although some studies had methodological flaws, a recent high-quality randomized controlled trial (RCT) conducted by Schiffman

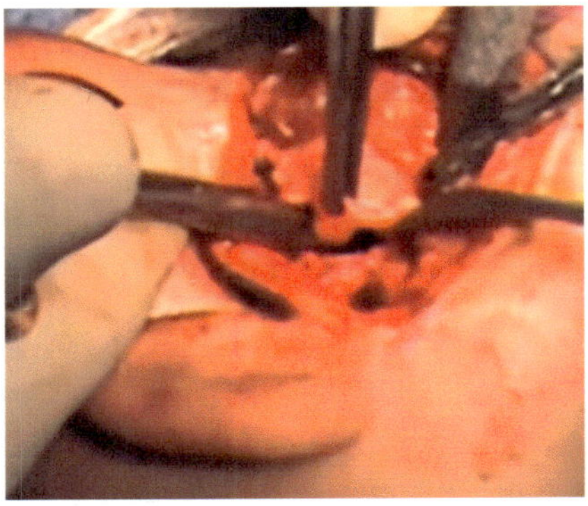

Figure 8.
Pretragic approach and capsular access for condylar TMJ intra-articular disorders.

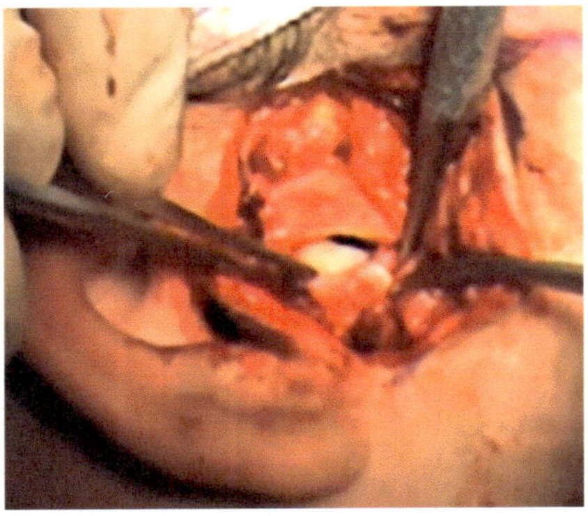

Figure 9.
Capsular opening in surgical treatment of intra-articular disorders.

et al. corroborated these results. The research indicated that surgical interventions such as arthroscopy and arthroplasty did not provide additional advantages for patients with disc dislocation without reduction and restricted mouth opening, in comparison with medical treatment or nonsurgical therapy [25, 26]. Across various parameters, such as TMJ pain intensity, frequency, mandibular range of motion, TMJ sounds, and chewing impairment, no significant differences were noted at the follow-up period [25].

Additionally, another review highlighted enhancements in TMD joint suffering following intra-articular hyaluronic acid (HA) injections and corticosteroids compared to placebo injections, although no comparisons were made with the conservative approach. The review found no data of differences between HA or plasma rich in growth factors (PRGF), low or medium molecular weight HA, one or two-needle hyaluronic acid injection techniques, or arthrocentesis with or without hyaluronic acid. Regarding orthodontics and occlusal adjustment, no evidence supports the effectiveness of occlusal modifications compared to placebo in the treatment and prevention of temporomandibular disorders. This includes occlusal positioning or equilibration through orthopedic, orthodontic, and prosthodontic methods. While occlusion plays a crucial role in chewing and should be approached carefully in maxillofacial practice, current studies do not encourage an etiological relationship in TMD pathophysiology [27].

3. Arthrocentesis

3.1 Technique

Murakami and colleagues [28] pioneered a systematic description of temporomandibular joint (TMJ) arthrocentesis, coining it the "manipulation technique followed by pumping and hydraulic pressure". The TMJ arthrocentesis discussed in this article represents a modification of the traditional method, involving the insertion of two needles into the upper joint space. This adaptation allows for extensive lavage of the joint, along with the capability for aspiration and injection [29]. The procedure, as described by the authors, is detailed below, along with practical insights. Before the procedure, preoperative drugs, including antibiotics, corticosteroids, and painkillers, are administered. The patient is positioned at a 45° incline or lying prone at 180°, with the head turned to the unaffected side to allow better access to the surgical field. After thorough disinfection of the target area, the points for needle insertion are marked on the skin, following the method suggested by McCain:

1. A line is drawn from the tragus midpoint to the lateral canthus.

2. Two points are marked to indicate the articular fossa localization and TMJ eminence. The glenoid fossa is represented by the posterior point and is located 12 millimeters from the tragus midpoint and two millimeters below the drawn line. Articular eminence is designated in the anterior point, situated 10 millimeters further along this line and 10 mm below it (**Figure 10**).

Besides the illustration, palpating the joint and fossa during the patient's movements, such as lower jaw motion in various directions, including mouth opening and contralateral movement, offers crucial insights into joint anatomy. Before the needle

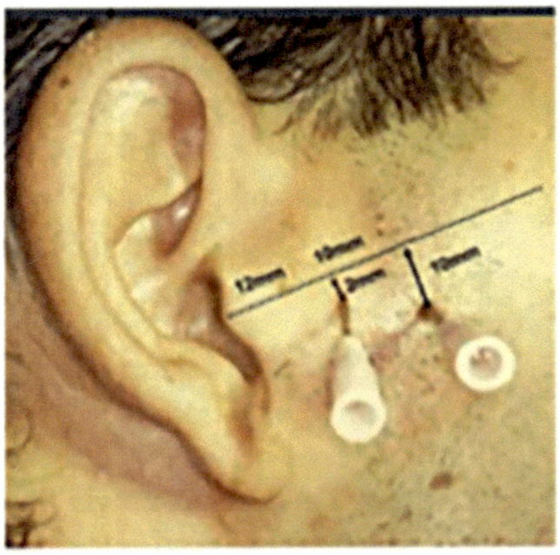

Figure 10.
For marking the entrance points in the upper compartment, a line is drawn from tragus midpoint to the lateral canthus. Subsequently, a posterior point designates the glenoid fossa, 10 millimeters from the tragus midpoint and two millimeters below this line. The anterior point denotes articular eminence, situated 10 millimeters further than the line and 5–10 millimeters below it.

insertion, a local anesthetic is applied pre-auricularly and subcutaneously where the needle will be inserted. Following this, a 19-gauge needle, connected to a one-milliliters syringe filled with Ringer solution, is carefully inserted into the superior zone of the articular fossa (**Figure 11**).

After the injection of Ringer's lactate, which is immediately aspirated to confirm that the needle is positioned in the upper joint space, 2–3 milliliters of lidocaine 0.5% is injected. This serves to distend upper joint space and surrounding tissues anesthesia. Following this, a second 19-gauge needle is inserted into the distended compartment near the articular eminence, facilitating a free flow of the Ringer's solution through the superior compartment (**Figures 12** and **13**).

The quantity of fluid traversing the joint is contingent on the procedural objective, distinguishing between tasks like disc release in anchored-disc phenomenon (ADP) and the elimination of deteriorated substances in osteoarthritis (OA). In instances of slow drainage, supplementary needles may be introduced into the expanded compartment to improve solution transport (**Figure 14**).

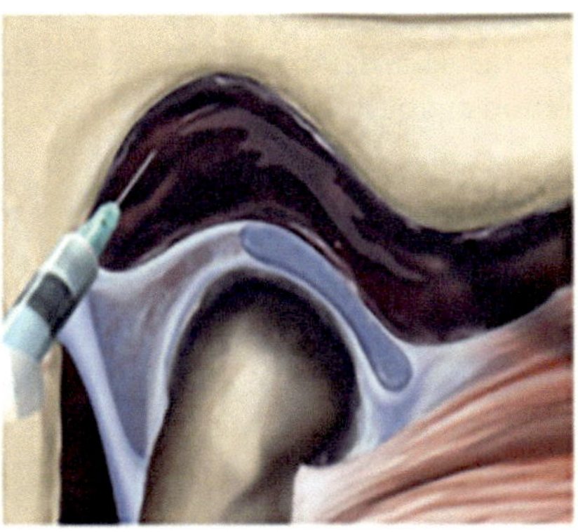

Figure 11.
The procedure consists of inserting a 19 G needle, which is attached to a one-milliliters syringe filled with Ringer solution, into the superior zone of the articular fossa. This action serves to distend the superior compartment.

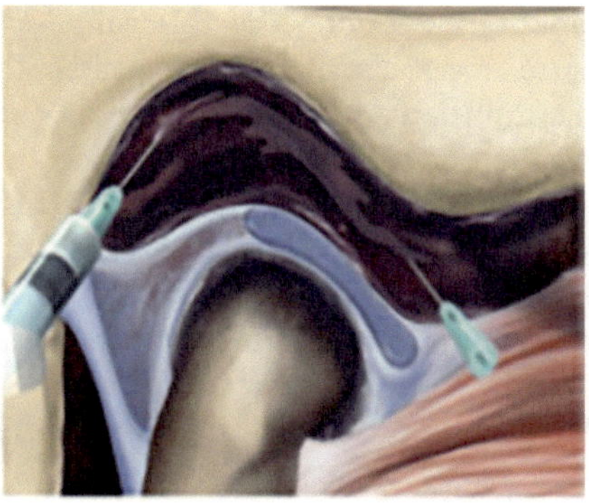

Figure 12.
A second 19-gauge needle is introduced into the distended superior compartment near the articular eminence.

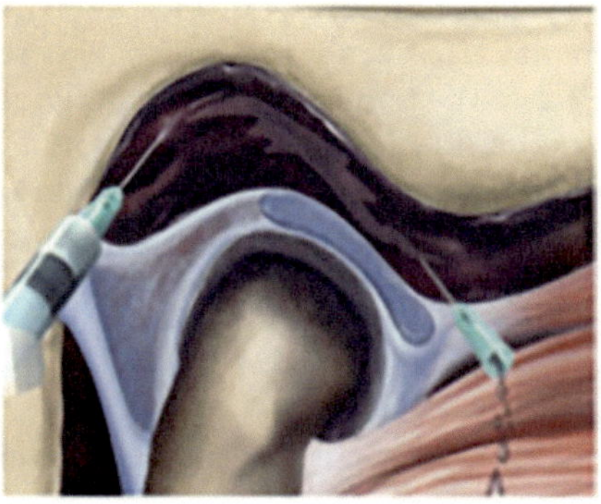

Figure 13.
A second 19-gauge needle is introduced into the expanded superior compartment around the articular eminence, facilitating the unimpeded flow of Ringer's lactate solution.

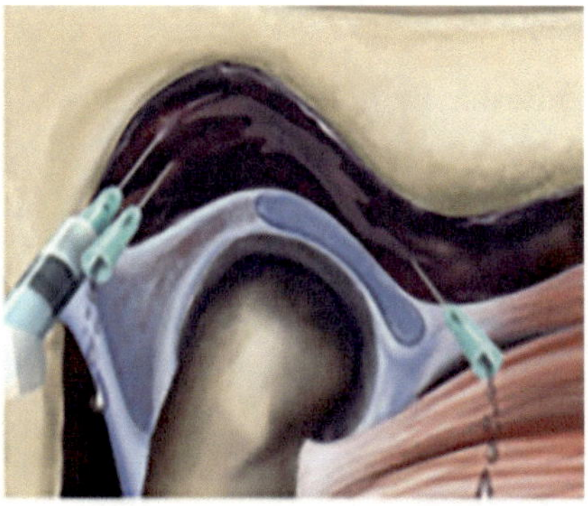

Figure 14.
In situations with sluggish additional outflow, introducing a third needle into the expanded compartment may be considered.

Various studies have explored the optimal volume of solution for arthrocentesis, suggesting amounts ranging from 100 mL to 400 mL, aiming for the elimination of detectable protein and bradykinin [30]. In difficult situations, another needle can be introduced in the posterior or in the superior zone. Following this, saline solution is injectied in the upper compartment to ensure proper distension and facilitate the procedure (**Figure 15**).

In challenging cases, a simplified approach can enhance accessibility by inserting the needle directly, approximately 90° in the eminence posterior aspect. This specific area is individuated when a contralateral mandibular shifting is performed, making it easier to locate and access during the procedure (**Figure 16a**).

There are several variants of the arthrocentesis technique, including a single-needle cannula technique by Nardini and a double needle cannula technique. Typically, one session is enough, but more intensive procedures involving five sessions/week have been documented. Various modifications in the execution of arthrocentesis have been reported [31].

After completing the procedure and removing one needle, medications such as steroids, opioids (like morphine, fentanyl, or tramadol), or HA intra-articular injection [32]. The appropriate HA molecular weight and its efficacy are still debated. Hyaluronic acid is not a lubricant, it is quickly degraded by the action of free radicals, thus it is important to remove inflammatory radicals through arthrocentesis before injecting HA. There has also been some controversy regarding the injection of platelet-rich plasma (PRP) into the temporomandibular joint alongside with arthrocentesis. Long-term studies should address concerns about PRP potentially promoting excessive bone growth or ankylosis [33]. Following this minimally invasive procedure, patients are usually monitored for about an hour. It is essential to view arthrocentesis as part of a broader treatment plan that includes an occlusal device, habits modification, and addressing any occlusal issues such as crossbite.

Contraindications for arthrocentesis include:

1. Locoregional and systemic infectious diseases (e.g., skin lesions, or herpetic infection, septic arthritis).

2. Locoregional neoplastic disorder.

3. Conditions affecting the skull base in the glenoid fossa region.

4. History of joint surgery.

5. Ankylosis causing limitation in mouth opening.

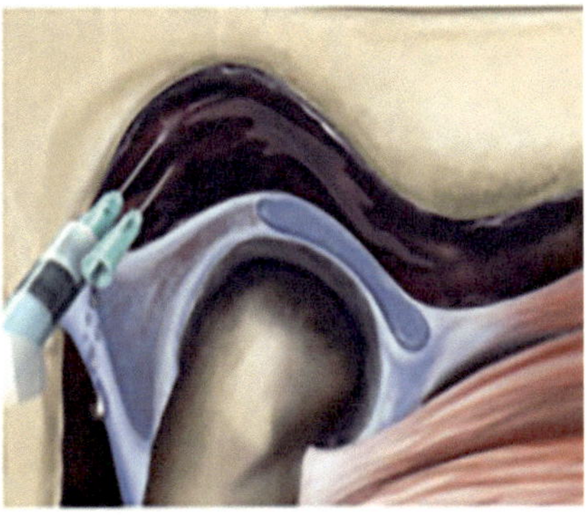

Figure 15.
In cases presenting technical challenges, the second needle can be inserted adjacent to the first, targeting the posterior compartment rather than the anterior one.

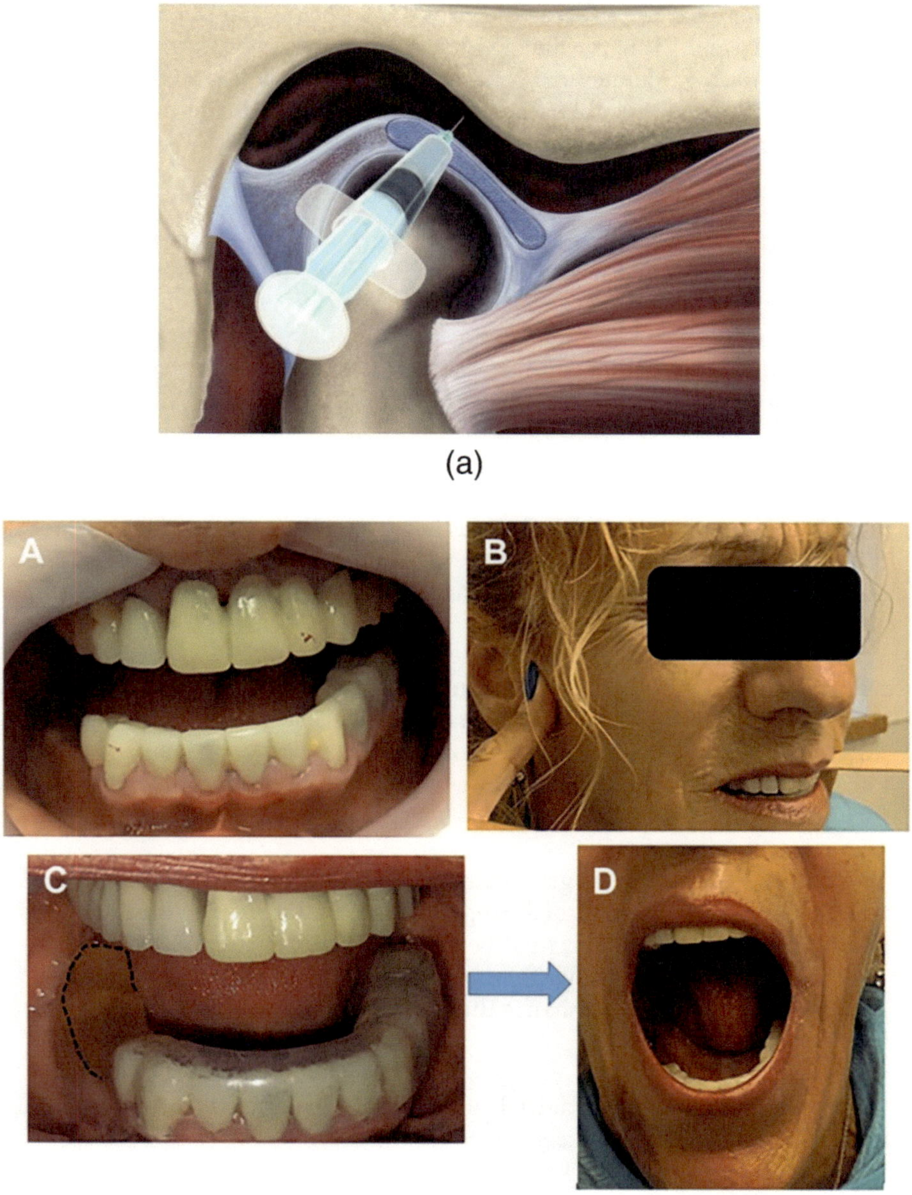

Figure 16.
(a) An alternative method for achieving straightforward access to the compartment is to insert a needle at approximately 90° on the posterior eminence part. This technique is particularly effective when the patient engages in contralateral mandibular shifting, as it helps to clearly identify the target area for the needle insertion. (b) A The patient undergoes 4.6–4.7 extraction and immediate implant loading without temporary prosthesis. B A sudden excess loading on the impaired right TMJ causes severe right TMJ suffering. C The application of an intra-occlusal device achieves load control and the correct occlusal height. TMJ arthrocentesis was performed D The immediate range of motion is shown.

Complications are uncommon and momentary. Indeed, facial paralysis can occur as a result of local anesthesia, and the infusion of saline solution could result in surrounding tissue swelling. Fortunately, these effects are self-resolving in 1 or

2 hours. While there have been rare reports of more serious complications, such as ear or brain injury and VII nerve damage, these evidence is significantly minimized when the established guidelines and protocols are respected. It is always important to follow best practices to ensure patient safety and comfort during and after the procedure [34, 35].

Tips:

- Performing local anesthesia in arthrocentesis procedures is essential for ensuring high patient compliance during the procedure. This approach helps to minimize discomfort while avoiding the need for unnecessary general anesthesia, which can carry additional risks and complications. By using local anesthesia, patients can remain more alert and comfortable, making the procedure smoother for both the patient and the healthcare provider.

- Joint clinical palpation is a core step in the procedure, as it allows the practitioner to accurately locate the appropriate insertion points for the needle. By feeling the joint and identifying marked points, the healthcare provider can ensure precise needle placement, which is essential for the success of the procedure. This careful approach helps to minimize discomfort and maximize the effectiveness of the treatment.

- Palpating the fossa while the condyle is moved contralaterally is a helpful technique. This movement allows the practitioner to better identify the anatomical landmarks and ensure accurate needle placement during the procedure. By feeling the changes in the joint position, the healthcare provider can enhance the precision of the arthrocentesis, leading to improved outcomes for the patient.

- Using 18 or 19 G needle is a great choice for arthrocentesis. These larger, rigid needles provide better control during the procedure, reducing the likelihood of bending or breaking. This rigidity is particularly beneficial when navigating the joint space, as it allows for more precise insertion and manipulation. Better needle control can enhance the overall effectiveness of the procedure and improve patient outcomes.

- Using one cc syringe for the initial entry point is an effective strategy to minimize distension due to an excess of fluid from seeping into the surrounding tissues. This approach allows for better control and precision when confirming the correct intra-articular location before proceeding with larger volumes. By ensuring that the needle is accurately placed within the joint space, you can enhance the success of the procedure and reduce the risk of complications.

- Suck-in effect is a valuable indicator that helps confirm the correct intra-articular location during arthrocentesis. When the needle is properly positioned within the joint space, the negative pressure can create a slight vacuum effect, drawing the syringe inward. This sensation is a helpful clue for the practitioner, indicating that they are in the right spot. Recognizing this effect can enhance the accuracy of the procedure and contribute to better outcomes for the patient.

- Ensure that all fluid introduced into the joint exits the joint to prevent intra and postoperative pain and swelling.

- In joints that are technically challenging, placing a second needle next to the first needle, parallel to it, can help improve the drainage of saline solution.
- Directly inserting the 1° needle at a 90° angle into the posterior slope of the eminence while the patient performs contralateral movements is an alternative approach.
- One needle soft pumping may assist in freeing the disc in case of adhesive forces causing adhesion to the temporal prominence.
- It is advisable that arthrocentesis is followed by load-biting control. For example, bite therapy, habit modification, and correction of occlusal issues such as cross-bite (**Figure 16b**).

3.2 Arthrocentesis: Mode of action

The impressive effectiveness of arthrocentesis has offered significant insights into TMJ function, dysfunction, and rehabilitation. Affected joints display synovial fluid that contains pain citokines, degraded enzimes, inflammation substances, pus if the infection is present, and bloody fluid in situations of hemarthrosis. These elements are detrimental to the joint, increasing internal loading, resulting in restricted function, discomfort, and misaligning pattern. Removing these substances through arthrocentesis alleviates suffering, reduces intra-articular pressure, and addresses the developed malocclusion. Arthrocentesis frees adhesions and separates the disc from the temporal cavity, allowing for unhindered disc movement. The combination of a released discal component, the removal of inflammatory reactive, and the decrease in intra-articular stress facilitates crucial functional rehabilitation essential for joint health [36].

Arthrocentesis has evolved into a significant diagnostic tool. Computer Tomography (CT) scan results do not consistently correlate with clinical signs, symptoms, or arthrocentesis reactions; therefore, they could not be the unique factor for a surgical operation decision [37].

Conversely, poor arthrocentesis outcome indicates evidence that TMJ surgery could be contemplated. In fact, arthrocentesis is often a precondition for TMJ surgical operations. Thus, if arthrocentesis is proven to be unsuccessful, it is reasonable to consider referring the patient for surgery.

In sum, arthrocentesis:

- Frees the disc and enhances sliding/function, crucial for joint integrity;
- Eliminates harmful substances from the joint, promoting a healthier environment;
- May alleviate joint pain, providing relief to the patient;
- Resolves malocclusion when caused by joint effusion;
- Eliminates increased intrinsic joint loading, reducing stress on the joint;
- Enables the revival of the lubrication system within the joint;
- Serves as a valuable diagnostic tool for assessing joint health and response.

However, It is important to emphasize that arthrocentesis should always be accompanied by joint loading management, which can be achieved through the use of bite therapy and diet modification, as well as the removal of occlusal issues impacting the joint. These accompanying measures contribute to the overall success and sustained benefits of the arthrocentesis procedure.

4. What do we evaluate? The role of arthrocentesis in various temporomandibular joint disorders (TMJD)

Arthrocentesis is a highly effective and enduring treatment method for managing pain and restricted range of motion [38].

4.1 Clicking joint

Constant clicking often stems from disc displacement (DD) in the TMJ. Interestingly, this displacement might occur without symptoms, present in over a third of joints in asymptomatic individuals. Conversely, normal disc positioning can exist in clicking joints [39]. The disc displacement typically results from joint overload, leading to lubrication compromise in the upper compartment. This disrupts disc sliding, weakens the condyle-disc relationship, and loosens ligaments attaching the disc to the condyle, facilitating displacement [40].

Arthrocentesis in constant clicking cases can enhance the displaced disc's sliding but does not aim to reposition it, thus the debate around its ability to eliminate these clicks. However, flushing the upper compartment often softens some clicks and even eliminates others, relieving the associated pain. Conversely, sporadic disc adherence to the fossa causing intermittent clicking can be managed by arthrocentesis and subsequent joint loading control. Extensive studies on arthrocentesis's long-term efficacy for clicking joints are still necessary [41].

4.2 Limited mouth opening

"Limited mouth opening" includes various disorders of diverse origins, that need specific attention:

- Disc displacement with or without intermittent locking.
- Anchored-disc phenomenon.
- Degenerative joint disease.

4.2.1 Disc displacement without reduction

When the disc undergoes displacement without returning to its original position, the sliding of the condyle is restricted, moderately impeding the mouth opening. Unless accompanied by pain, this condition might often go unnoticed.

Symptomatic disc displacement without reduction manifests with a restricted mouth opening, typically ranging from 25 to 30 mm. It usually involves a history of clicking. Pain arises during forced mouth opening and loading of the affected joint, caused by excessive strain on the highly sensitive retro-discal tissue that has not yet been adopted.

Radiographs and CT scans reveal evidence of limited condylar sliding, while arthrography and magnetic resonance imaging (MRI), display the disc positioned in front of the condyle in both closed and open mouth positions.

It has been observed that arthrocentesis reduces limitations and pain resulting from disc dislocation. Although it does not reposition the disc, it facilitates freer sliding in the upper compartment, thereby improving mouth opening [42].

4.2.2 Anchored-disc phenomenon

The anchored-disc phenomenon (**Figure 17**) presents with a sudden and persistently restricted mouth opening, typically ranging between 10 and 25 mm, accompanied by deviation toward the affected side. Movements toward the opposite side are limited, and upon protrusion, the mandible tends to deviate toward the affected side. Unlike other conditions, a history of clicking is not necessary for the diagnosis. While pain during joint loading is uncommon, forced mouth opening triggers pain in the affected joint.

In long-lasting cases of anchored-disc phenomenon, the distinctive clinical features may become less pronounced. Radiographs and CT scans reveal the absence of sliding in the TMJ with the condyle, which usually rotates under the disc, displaying atypical structure [43].

In MRI, the disc seems attached to the articular prominence, and the condyle moves under the disc. The existence of adhesive forces between the disc and fossa has been suggested to explain the limitation of disc movement [44]. Overloading of the joint reduces joint lubrication, producing cohesive forces between the disc and the fossa [43]. Forcibly opening it is not advisable as it might result in stretching and shearing of the joint's ligaments. Arthrocentesis immediately counteracts these cohesive forces, facilitating a smooth and natural opening of the mouth. Arthrocentesis always accompanies joint loading control by employing an occlusal device, implementing a soft diet, eliminating any occlusal hazard, and utilizing physiotherapy without joint loading (physical therapy, certainly not recommended while the disc is lodged, should be extensively used after disc release) [45].

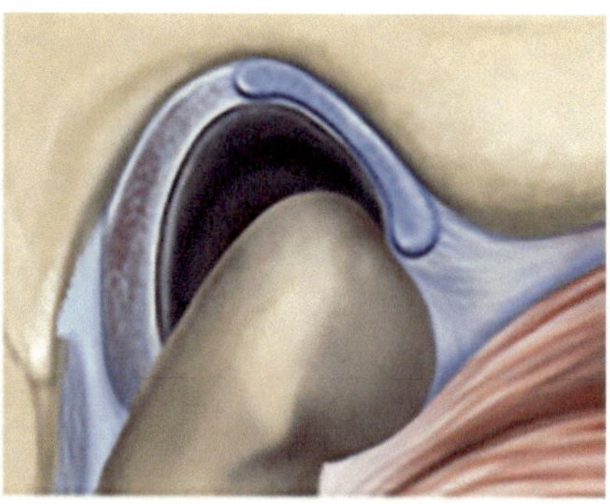

Figure 17.
In the anterior disc position (ADP), the disc adheres to the articular eminence through adhesive forces, while the condyle remains constrained posteriorly.

4.2.3 Open-lock versus TMJ condyle dislocation

Open-lock is an unexpected incapacity of mouth closing and it is typically resolved by patient's manipulation. The extent of opening in the open-lock is not pronounced as in dislocation of the condyle and the value is 25–30 mm. In X-rays and CT, in the open lock, the condyle position is under the prominence. The open lock is caused by insufficient lubrification, which increases the contact of disc and prominence. Normally, the disc moves in coordination along the condyle, but when it lags behind, the condyle slides underneath and before the disc. This displacement prevents the disc from returning to its proper position within the fossa, resulting in a mouth that remains constantly open. In managing open locks, nonsurgical methods are usually efficacious. If not, irrigation of the upper compartment can restore the movement of the disc, allowing synchronized movement of both the disc and the condyle. Preventing the condyle from advancing beyond the disc leads to infrequent instances of long-term recurrence [46].

4.3 Osteoarthritis

Temporomandibular joint osteoarthritis (TMJ OA) shows cartilage breakdown, subchondral bone hardening, and ongoing inflammation in the synovial tissue (**Figure 18A**). Unlike the hip or knee, it tends to manifest across all age groups [38], following a bell curve rather than correlating with age. We view TMJ OA as a joint's adaptive progression: when the joint adjusts, we note structural alterations, yet the joint stays symptom-free. But when the joint fails to adapt, it becomes symptomatic, leading to one or more issues such as joint pain, restricted movement, and occlusal modifications (**Figure 18B**).

The aim of treating symptomatic OA is to restore the joint to a more adaptable condition [47]. Interestingly, arthrocentesis brings about substantial improvement in 82% of patients, even though it does not alter the actual joint structure. This action helps return the joint to its adaptable state, eliminating the necessity for further surgical intervention. The development of TMJ OA remains a subject of debate; likewise, there's ongoing discussion regarding whether TMJ OA is an isolated incident

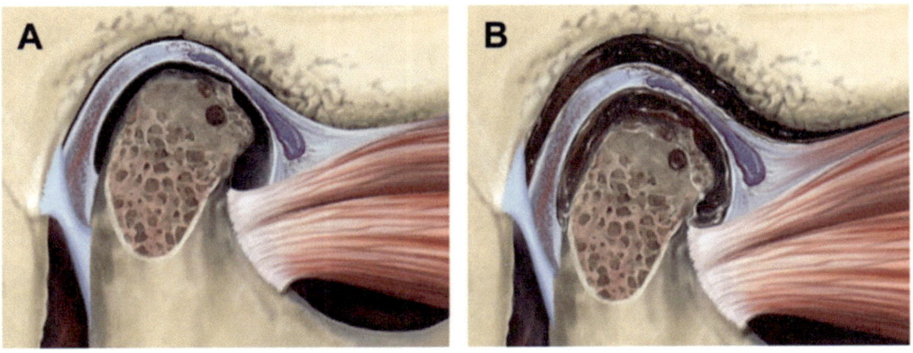

Figure 18.
Osteoarthritis of the temporomandibular joint is distinguished by **A** *The deterioration of cartilage, sclerosis of the subchondral bone, presence of cysts, cortical boundary erosion, formation of osteophytes, reduction of intra-articular space, and a perforated, irritated disc;* **B** *Inflammatory intra-articular fluids could expand the intra-articular zone, which may cause disruptions in occlusion and lead to malocclusion.*

or the culmination of an internal derangement process. Another quandary revolves around whether OA commences with cartilage collapse penetrating the subchondral bone, as commonly believed, or if it initiates with subchondral bone hardening followed by cartilage collapse, as indicated in documented cases. In the acute phase, patients might experience symptoms, including stiffness in the morning, restricted mouth opening—sometimes accompanied by localized joint pain—and discomfort in biting especially on the contralateral TMJ. Occasionally, patients do not realize they are evolving in a gradual, painless limitation in the maxilla-mandibular opening. Crepitus, which may or may not be accompanied by clicking sounds, could appear in TMJ movements [48]. RM studies of arthritic joints can show various levels of changes. In more advanced scenarios, common findings include cortical erosion, reduced intra-articular area, formation of osteophyte, cortical cysts, and disc perforation.

By discal freeing and removing factors contributing to discomfort, we enable mobilization, which we see as the primary avenue to recovery. This result heavily relies on joint movements that generate the necessary fluctuating pressures within the joint, acting akin to a pump. This means that the restoration of oxygenation, nutrient supply, waste elimination, and joint lubrication is anticipated to reestablish the joint's self-correction.

Interestingly, there is a lack of substantial correlation between the patient's observable signs and symptoms and the findings on X-rays. Additionally, no significant correlation has been found in radiographic severity findings compared with arthrocentesis results. In simpler terms, the clinical symptoms and the degree of imaging changes are not reliable predictors of the success of arthrocentesis [37].

This underscores the significance of arthrocentesis as a crucial diagnostic tool that determines the necessity for further surgical procedures.

There are several notable points regarding TMJ OA:

- The occurrence of TMJ OA does not escalate with age.
- Arthrocentesis proves highly effective in managing pain and restoring function in symptomatic TMJ OA cases, preventing the need for more invasive surgical measures.
- The success rate of arthrocentesis in TMJ OA patients is not influenced by age.
- There is a lack of substantial connection between a patient's observable signs and symptoms and the findings seen on X-rays. Similarly, there is no clear association between the severity of radiographic observations and the outcomes of arthrocentesis.
- Unlike long bones, the TMJ retains its ability to remodel due to the presence of proliferative mesenchymal cells, allowing conservative treatments to yield positive results regardless of age.
- Managing the joint's loading is pivotal in the rehabilitation process.
- The patient should diligently practice consistent physiotherapy, with a focus on avoiding joint overloading. This approach becomes more effective and safer after the patient has undergone arthrocentesis.

4.4 Inflammatory illness, hemarthrosis, and infection issues

TMJ hemarthrosis following jaw injury presents with the patient reporting painful swelling concentrated in the impacted joint and discomfort in their bite alignment [49]. Typically, there is restricted mouth opening, often accompanied by a shift toward the affected side, limited lateral movements to both right and left, and constrained protrusion that inclines toward the affected area. An open bite is commonly identified on the impacted side. Trans-cranial imaging, when the mouth is closed, typically exhibits an expansion of the space within the joint.

Immediate attention is crucial for addressing this condition, aiming to remove the blood and lower intra-articular pressure through arthrocentesis or intensive physiotherapy along with relieving joint stress to prevent potential joint damage and subsequent functional issues. Additionally, considering analgesics, anti-inflammatory medications, and antibiotics is advisable. It is important to note that inexperienced examiners might overlook a non-fractured condyle following trauma, leading to an inadequate diagnosis. Undetected TMJ hemarthrosis could result in the formation of fibrous adhesions.

Various systemic conditions like rheumatoid arthritis, idiopathic juvenile arthritis, psoriatic arthritis, and familial Mediterranean fever, among others, can also contribute to TMJ pain and dysfunction. While the source of the symptoms is systemic, local treatments like arthrocentesis can complement overall treatment approaches. If necessary, the procedure can be repeated. It is important to emphasize that alongside arthrocentesis, load control, physiotherapy, and addressing any existing occlusal risks should always be incorporated.

5. Future perspectives

5.1 Injectable-platelet rich fibrin

Platelet rich fibrin (PRF), as a second-generation platelet concentrate, offers several advantages over platelet-rich plasma (PRP). Its preparation does not require external additives, minimizing the risk of adverse patient reactions. The technology involved in PRF preparation is straightforward and achieved through a single-step centrifugation process [50]. Additionally, PRF naturally undergoes slow polymerization during centrifugation. This natural polymerization, devoid of thrombin, results in an enhanced and more malleable fibrin network, facilitating cytokine liberation and cell resettlement [50]. Gradual polymerization of the fibrin component in PRF ensures the core integration of resident-cytokines of the platelet components and sugar cuffs into the fibrin complex. This gradual release of cytokines during fibrin matrix remodeling creates an environment conducive to the healing process [50, 51]. Studies indicate that injectable PRF (I-PRF) obtained through low-speed centrifugation consistently releases higher levels of inflammatory cells, platelets, and growth factors [52]. Moreover, this sustained release of elevated growth factors can more effectively stimulate cartilage regeneration compared to PRP [53, 54]. The mechanism by which PRF treats TMD likely involves joint regulation through platelet-release mediators and fibrin matrix. Similar to PRP, platelet-release mediators in PRF inhibit inflammation, support chondrocyte proliferation, and aid in cartilage repair. The unique three-dimensional reticular structure of the fibrin matrix supports cell migration, enabling PRF to gradually release growth factors and cytokines, thereby extending the action duration of these factors and enhancing the treatment's effectiveness. Currently, injectable PRF remains the sole form of PRF utilized in TMD treatment.

Injectable-platelet fibrin (I-PRF) retains growth factors and cells within the joint space, ensuring their sustained release for prolonged periods, enhancing TMJ functional activity, and providing relief from pain [55]. This sustained state is believed to endure for 12 months, effectively reinstating intra-articular balance. The resulting absence of a standardized method for practicing PRP could result in variations in its configuration and curative effectiveness. Diverse arrangement techniques could result in the presence of leukocytes in PRP, and the clinical outcomes and cellular impacts of leukocyte-rich or -poor PRP remain a topic of controversy [56].

In contrast, the composition and preparation of I-PRF tend to be more refined compared to the complexities associated with PRP. Currently, PRF offers more advantages and seems to be a superior choice. However, further research is necessary to substantiate the long-term efficacy of PRF. The maturity in the composition and preparation of I-PRF makes it a promising avenue for TMJ treatment, emphasizing its potential over conventional PRP methods.

PRP-HA blending shows potential owing to a harmonized activity. The regenerative attributes of the Platelet Rich Fibrin component facilitate healing and restoration of the tissue and the lubricating and anti-inflammatory effects of HA provide joint well-being and suffering alleviation. Merging Platelet Rich Fibrin and hyaluronic acid could produce synergism in action, and pain mitigation function optimization in TMD patients [57]. Cytokines and growth factors present in PRP might amplify HA's anti-inflammatory effects, fostering a more stable and balanced response of immune system within the joint.

Concurrently, lubricating action of hyaluronic acid can improve the allocation of PRP restorative components in TMJ space, hypothetically protracting their positive impacts [58].

Additionally, understanding the timing and dosage considerations for this combined treatment is crucial for its effectiveness. By determining the optimal administration schedule and dosage levels for both PRP and HA, we can better comprehend their cumulative impact on pain perception.

This combined approach faces various facets of pain manifestation, encompassing flogosis, tissue impairment, and compromised lubrication. As a result, it could offer a more inclusive treatment to suffering alleviation compared to individual managements [59].

5.2 Platelet-rich plasma (PRP) and hyaluronic acid (HA)

Combination therapies, such as the fusion of PRP and HA, are utilized in regenerative medicine and joint pain management, catering to a wide array of medical conditions [60]. The specific dosage, duration of treatment, and administration protocols depend on various factors, including the patient's condition and the guidance of the physician. PRP dosages are tailored concerning the extracted blood volume and the chosen concentration of platelet component, usually planning for a five-fold spread over the normal level. Usually, PRP is injected in volumes ranging from three to five milliliters per TMJ site.

For HA, dosage level depends on the HA molecular specificity and treatment site, with typical injections spanning 1–3 milliliters per joint or focal point. Treatment regimens usually involve several injections, typically 3 or 5 sittings spread over a seven-twelve day interval. Succeeding additional injection might be required for continuous suffering alleviation and TMJ function, ranging from some months to 12 months, and so on. These infiltrations are usually injected directly in the impaired zone by a qualified surgeon, under ultrasound view. PRP-HA synergical action requires supplementary examination by clinical reports assessing their united improvement in suffering and function, and their outcomes according to patient and surgeon satisfaction after treatment. Those studies should offer a precious understanding of optimal medicating, timing, and approach to improve the outcomes of PRP-HA use in TMJ minimally invasive management.

5.3 Tissue engineering involving stem cells

Tissue engineering involving stem cells presents a compelling and promising avenue for regenerative therapy. Stem cells primarily originate from two sources: embryonic stem cells (ESCs) and adult stem cells, notably mesenchymal stem cells (MSCs), which are extensively utilized in TMJ treatments. These cells are employed in repairing damaged tissues or those with impaired function. Their role is to replace and restore normal tissue physiology while also regulating the inflammatory process. By doing so, they aim to reduce painful symptoms, and halt the progressive degeneration of cartilage and subchondral bone, ultimately aiding in the restoration of TMJ function [61].

Due to their multipotent nature and ability to be obtained from various sites like muscle, bone, umbilical cord, fat tissue, dermal component, blood, dental pulp, and synovial fluid, stem cells possess the capability to differentiate into diverse cell types, including adipocytes, osteocytes, and chondrocytes. Depending on the extent of joint damage, these stem cells play a crucial role in tissue repair and regeneration while also suppressing inflammation and modulating the immune response. In the initial stages of joint osteoarthritis, they exhibit protective, homeostatic, and regenerative functions, while in more advanced stages, they contribute to delaying tissue degeneration. Chondrocytes and osteoblasts were the primary cell types differentiated from stem cells for in vitro analysis [61].

The activation of Interleukin-1β (IL-1β) plays a significant role as a risk factor in temporomandibular joint osteoarthritis (TMJOA). TMJOA represents the most severe form of temporomandibular disorders, characterized by damage to the condylar cartilage and abnormal sclerosis in the subchondral bone [62]. Synovial inflammation is a key element in the pathogenesis of osteoarthritis (OA), and pro-inflammatory cytokines are hypothesized to be pivotal in TMJOA development. Interleukin-1β (IL-1β), recognized as one of the most potent pro-inflammatory cytokines, is the primary cytokine produced in response to excessive joint loading. IL-1β prompts an increase in the generation of reactive oxygen species (ROS), leading to the production of numerous peroxides and hydroxyl radicals that can directly harm the articular cartilage [63]. Patients with OA typically exhibit elevated levels of IL-1β in various areas, including the synovial fluid, synovial membrane, cartilage, and the subchondral bone layer (**Figure 19**).

Thus far, clinical trials employing anti-cytokine therapies for OA have shown varying outcomes. In recent years, gene chip technology has been extensively utilized to explore the molecular mechanisms underlying disease progression.

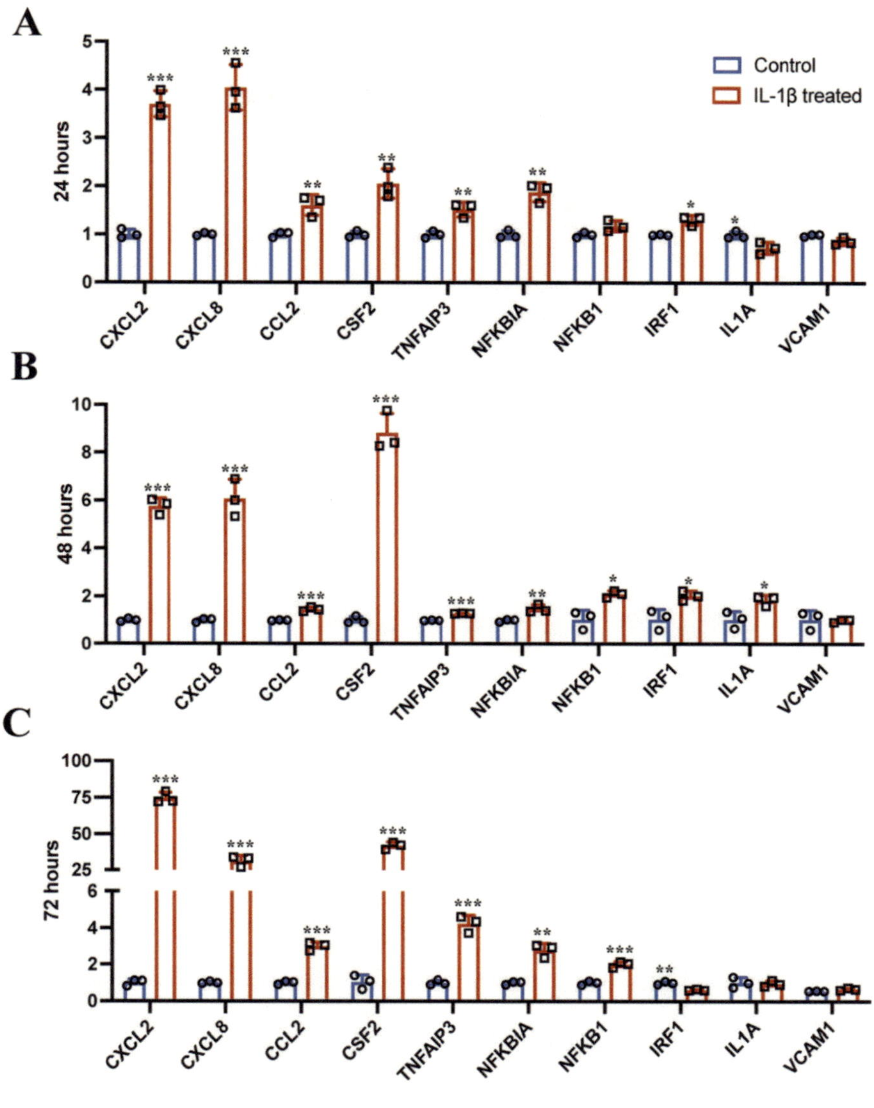

Figure 19.
The expression of inflammatory factors in mscs stimulated with il-1beta after different time points.

This particular study identified 200 DEGs (differentially expressed genes) [64], comprising 168 mRNA and 32 LNCRNA (**Figure 20**), and pinpointed the top 10 hub genes: CXCL8, CCL2, CXCL2, NFKBIA, CSF2, IL1A, IRF1, VCAM1, NFKB1, TNFAIP3 [65].

Among these, CXCL8, CCL2, and CXCL2 represent chemokines that influence the immune system and the release of matrix-degrading enzymes during cartilage remodeling and deterioration in OA. Notably, increased expression of CXCL8 (also known as IL-8) has been observed in OA synovial fluid. CCL2, a chemokine ligand, is expressed in chondrocytes, osteoblasts, and synoviocytes, contributing to bone metabolism and playing a role in OA. Monocytes recruited *via* CCL2 further fuel inflammation and tissue damage in OA [66].

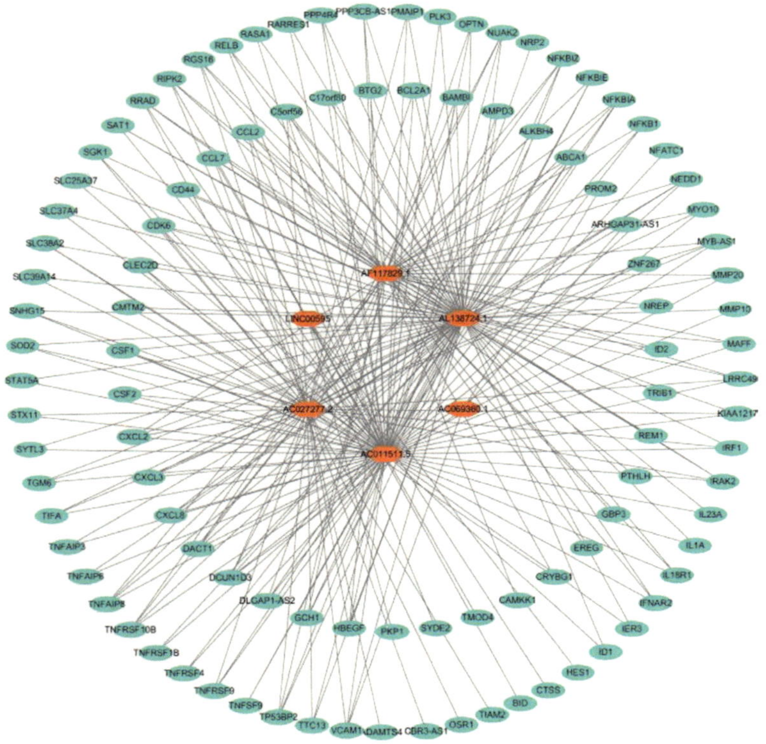

Figure 20.
LNCRNA-MRNA co-expression network.

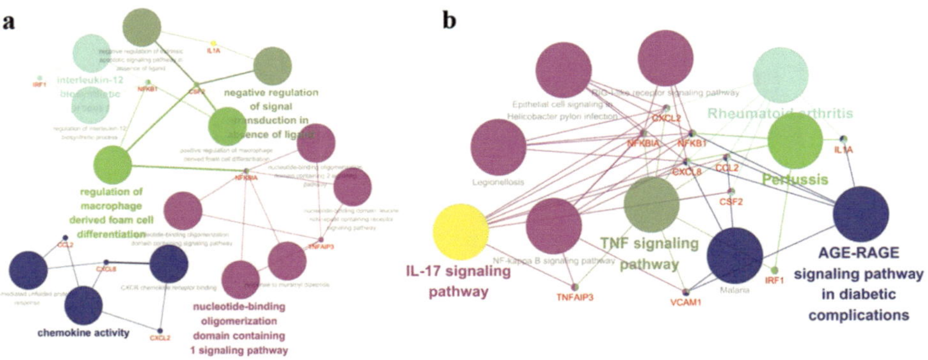

Figure 21.
A Analysis of hub genes B analysis of patways.

The pro-inflammatory and catabolic impacts of IL-1β are orchestrated through the activation of diverse signaling pathways, including the TNF signaling pathway, NF-κB signaling pathway, NOD-like receptors signaling pathway, and cytokine-cytokine-receptor interaction [67]. TNF is pivotal in instigating the inflammatory cascade and can act in conjunction with IL-1β or independently, initiating and perpetuating inflammation. TNF-α activation of the NF-κB signaling pathway induces the manifestation of various genes of inflammation such as iNOS -COX2, chemokines, and supplies MMP1, MMP9, MMP13, and ADAMTS4 upregulation (**Figures 21** and **22**) [68].

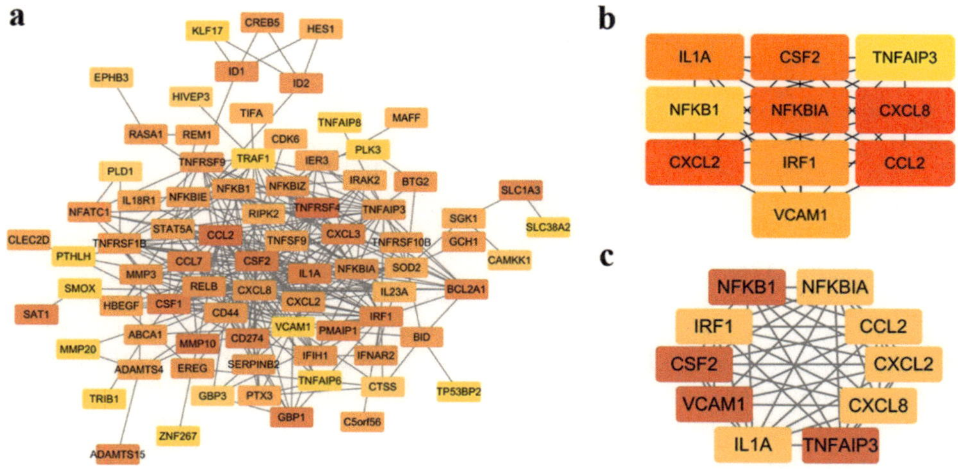

Figure 22.
Protein–Protein interaction network: Figure a shows that the module contained 152 nodes and 320 edges and the average nodal degree was 4.21. Figure b shows that the top hub genes identified were CXCL8, CCL2, CXCL2, NFKBIA, CSF2, IL1A, IRF1, VCAM1, NFKB1, and TNFAIP3. Figure c shows the core subnetwork constructed by these genes (maybe the key nodes in the protein protein interaction (PPI) network).

In summary, although some causes of TMJOA, like genetic factors and aging, are inevitable, we might influence the disease by targeting cellular communication within the TMJOA network. Understanding the intricate dependencies in this network could pave the way for targeted therapies using cytokines, antibodies, and other recombinant biological factors to disrupt the self-perpetuating cycle of the disease process.

Author details

Mario Santagata, Ciro Emiliano Boschetti, Giuseppe Colella, Carmelo Consiglio, Roberta Magliulo, Roberta Sivo, Davide Morlando, Annalisa Pollice, David Guida, Ivo Ferrieri, Salvatore D'Amato, Luigi Rugge, Gianpaolo Tartaro and Fabrizio Chirico*
Maxillofacial Surgery Unit, University of Campania "Luigi Vanvitelli", Naples, Italy

*Address all correspondence to: fabriziochirico@hotmail.com

References

[1] Kapos FP, Exposto FG, Oyarzo JF, Durham J. Temporomandibular disorders: A review of current concepts in aetiology, diagnosis and management. Oral Surgery. 2020;**13**(4):321-334. DOI: 10.1111/ors.12473

[2] Bair E, Gaynor S, Slade GD, et al. Identification of clusters of individuals relevant to temporomandibular disorders and other chronic pain conditions: The OPPERA study. Pain. 2016;**157**(6):1266-1278. DOI: 10.1097/j.pain.0000000000000518

[3] Slade GD, Sanders AE, Bair E, et al. Preclinical episodes of orofacial pain symptoms and their association with health care behaviors in the OPPERA prospective cohort study. Pain. 2013;**154**(5):750-760. DOI: 10.1016/j.pain.2013.01.014

[4] Meloto CB, Bortsov AV, Bair E, et al. Modification of COMT-dependent pain sensitivity by psychological stress and sex. Pain. 2016;**157**(4):858-867. DOI: 10.1097/j.pain.0000000000000449

[5] Helkimo M. Studies on function and dysfunction of the masticatory system. II. Index for anamnestic and clinical dysfunction and occlusal state. Svensk Tandläkare Tidskrift. 1974;**67**(2):101-121

[6] Manfredini D, Winocur E, Ahlberg J, Guarda-Nardini L, Lobbezoo F. Psychosocial impairment in temporomandibular disorders patients. RDC/TMD axis II findings from a multicentre study. Journal of Dentistry. 2010;**38**(10):765-772. DOI: 10.1016/j.jdent.2010.06.007

[7] Lövgren A, Visscher CM, Häggman-Henrikson B, Lobbezoo F, Marklund S, Wänman A. Validity of three screening questions (3Q/TMD) in relation to the DC/TMD. Journal of Oral Rehabilitation. 2016;**43**(10):729-736. DOI: 10.1111/joor.12428

[8] Lövgren A, Parvaneh H, Lobbezoo F, Häggman-Henrikson B, Wänman A, Visscher CM. Diagnostic accuracy of three screening questions (3Q/TMD) in relation to the DC/TMD in a specialized orofacial pain clinic. Acta Odontologica Scandinavica. 2018;**76**(6):380-386. DOI: 10.1080/00016357.2018.1439528

[9] Treede RD, Rief W, Barke A, et al. Chronic pain as a symptom or a disease: The IASP classification of chronic pain for the international classification of diseases (ICD-11). Pain. 2019;**160**(1):19-27. DOI: 10.1097/j.pain.0000000000001384

[10] Nicholas M, Vlaeyen JWS, Rief W, et al. The IASP classification of chronic pain for ICD-11: Chronic primary pain. Pain. 2019;**160**(1):28-37. DOI: 10.1097/j.pain.0000000000001390

[11] Dworkin SF, LeResche L. Research diagnostic criteria for temporomandibular disorders: Review, criteria, examinations and specifications, critique. Journal of Craniomandibular Disorders. 1992;**6**(4):301-355

[12] Schiffman E, Ohrbach R, Truelove E, et al. Diagnostic criteria for temporomandibular disorders (DC/TMD) for clinical and research applications: Recommendations of the international RDC/TMD consortium network* and orofacial pain special interest group†. Journal of Oral and Facial Pain and Headache. 2014;**28**(1):6-27. DOI: 10.11607/jop.1151

[13] Gonzalez YM, Schiffman E, Gordon SM, et al. Development of a

brief and effective temporomandibular disorder pain screening questionnaire: Reliability and validity. Journal of the American Dental Association (1939). 2011;**142**(10):1183-1191. DOI: 10.14219/jada.archive.2011.0088

[14] Ceusters W, Michelotti A, Raphael KG, Durham J, Ohrbach R. Perspectives on next steps in classification of oro-facial pain - part 1: Role of ontology. Journal of Oral Rehabilitation. 2015;**42**(12):926-941. DOI: 10.1111/joor.12336

[15] Nixdorf DR, Drangsholt MT, Ettlin DA, et al. Classifying orofacial pains: A new proposal of taxonomy based on ontology. Journal of Oral Rehabilitation. 2012;**39**(3):161-169. DOI: 10.1111/j.1365-2842.2011.02247.x

[16] Chantaracherd P, John MT, Hodges JS, Schiffman EL. Temporomandibular joint disorders' impact on pain, function, and disability. Journal of Dental Research. 2015;**94**(Suppl. 3):79S-86S. DOI: 10.1177/0022034514565793

[17] Meloto CB, Slade GD, Lichtenwalter RN, et al. Clinical predictors of persistent temporomandibular disorder in people with first-onset temporomandibular disorder: A prospective case-control study. Journal of the American Dental Association (1939). 2019;**150**(7):572-581.e10. DOI: 10.1016/j.adaj.2019.03.023

[18] Durham J, Al-Baghdadi M, Baad-Hansen L, et al. Self-management programmes in temporomandibular disorders: Results from an international Delphi process. Journal of Oral Rehabilitation. 2016;**43**(12):929-936. DOI: 10.1111/joor.12448

[19] List T, Axelsson S. Management of TMD: Evidence from systematic reviews and meta-analyses. Journal of Oral Rehabilitation. 2010;**37**(6):430-451. DOI: 10.1111/j.1365-2842.2010.02089.x

[20] Häggman-Henrikson B, Alstergren P, Davidson T, et al. Pharmacological treatment of oro-facial pain - health technology assessment including a systematic review with network meta-analysis. Journal of Oral Rehabilitation. 2017;**44**(10):800-826. DOI: 10.1111/joor.12539

[21] Haviv Y, Rettman A, Aframian D, Sharav Y, Benoliel R. Myofascial pain: An open study on the pharmacotherapeutic response to stepped treatment with tricyclic antidepressants and gabapentin. Journal of Oral and Facial Pain and Headache. 2015;**29**(2):144-151. DOI: 10.11607/ofph.1408

[22] Aggarwal VR, Fu Y, Main CJ, Wu J. The effectiveness of self-management interventions in adults with chronic orofacial pain: A systematic review, meta-analysis and meta-regression. European Journal of Pain. 2019;**23**(5):849-865. DOI: 10.1002/ejp.1358

[23] Shimada A, Ishigaki S, Matsuka Y, et al. Effects of exercise therapy on painful temporomandibular disorders. Journal of Oral Rehabilitation. 2019;**46**(5):475-481. DOI: 10.1111/joor.12770

[24] Ceusters W, Nasri-Heir C, Alnaas D, Cairns BE, Michelotti A, Ohrbach R. Perspectives on next steps in classification of oro-facial pain - part 3: Biomarkers of chronic oro-facial pain - from research to clinic. Journal of Oral Rehabilitation. 2015;**42**(12):956-966. DOI: 10.1111/joor.12324

[25] Schiffman EL, Velly AM, Look JO, et al. Effects of four treatment strategies for temporomandibular joint closed

lock. International Journal of Oral and Maxillofacial Surgery. 2014;**43**(2):217-226. DOI: 10.1016/j.ijom.2013.07.744

[26] Wroclawski C, Mediratta JK, Fillmore WJ. Recent advances in temporomandibular joint surgery. Medicina (Kaunas). 2023;**59**(8):1409

[27] Ferreira N, Masterson D, Lopes de Lima R, et al. Efficacy of viscosupplementation with hyaluronic acid in temporomandibular disorders: A systematic review. Journal of Cranio-Maxillo-Facial Surgery. 2018;**46**(11):1943-1952. DOI: 10.1016/j.jcms.2018.08.007

[28] Murakami KI, Iizuka T, Matsuki M, Ono T. Recapturing the persistent anteriorly displaced disk by mandibular manipulation after pumping and hydraulic pressure to the upper joint cavity of the temporomandibular joint. Cranio. 1987;**5**(1):17-24. DOI: 10.1080/08869634.1987.11678169

[29] Nitzan DW, Dolwick MF, Martinez GA. Temporomandibular joint arthrocentesis: A simplified treatment for severe, limited mouth opening. Journal of Oral and Maxillofacial Surgery. 1991;**49**(11):1163-1170. DOI: 10.1016/0278-2391(91)90409-f

[30] Kaneyama K, Segami N, Nishimura M, Sato J, Fujimura K, Yoshimura H. The ideal lavage volume for removing bradykinin, interleukin-6, and protein from the temporomandibular joint by arthrocentesis. Journal of Oral and Maxillofacial Surgery. 2004;**62**(6):657-661. DOI: 10.1016/j.joms.2003.08.031

[31] Guarda-Nardini L, Tito R, Staffieri A, Beltrame A. Treatment of patients with arthrosis of the temporomandibular joint by infiltration of sodium hyaluronate: A preliminary study. European Archives of Oto-Rhino-Laryngology. 2002;**259**(5):279-284. DOI: 10.1007/s00405-002-0456-z

[32] Bergstrand S, Ingstad HK, Møystad A, Bjørnland T. Long-term effectiveness of arthrocentesis with and without hyaluronic acid injection for treatment of temporomandibular joint osteoarthritis. Journal of Oral Science. 2019;**61**(1):82-88. DOI: 10.2334/josnusd.17-0423

[33] Hancı M, Karamese M, Tosun Z, Aktan TM, Duman S, Savaci N. Intra-articular platelet-rich plasma injection for the treatment of temporomandibular disorders and a comparison with arthrocentesis. Journal of Cranio-Maxillo-Facial Surgery. 2015;**43**(1):162-166. DOI: 10.1016/j.jcms.2014.11.002

[34] Nogueira EFC, Lemos CAA, Vasconcellos RJH, Moraes SLD, Vasconcelos BCE, Pellizzer EP. Does arthroscopy cause more complications than arthrocentesis in patients with internal temporomandibular joint disorders? Systematic review and meta-analysis. The British Journal of Oral and Maxillofacial Surgery. 2021;**59**(10):1166-1173. DOI: 10.1016/j.bjoms.2021.05.007

[35] Carroll TA, Smith K, Jakubowski J. Extradural haematoma following temporomandibular joint arthrocentesis and lavage. British Journal of Neurosurgery. 2000;**14**(2):152-154. DOI: 10.1080/02688690050004633

[36] Eliav E, Teich S, Nitzan D, et al. Facial arthralgia and myalgia: Can they be differentiated by trigeminal sensory assessment? Pain. 2003;**104**(3):481-490. DOI: 10.1016/S0304-3959(03)00077-0

[37] Nitzan DW, Svidovsky J, Zini A, Zadik Y. Effect of Arthrocentesis on symptomatic osteoarthritis of the temporomandibular joint and analysis

of the effect of preoperative clinical and radiologic features. Journal of Oral and Maxillofacial Surgery. 2017;**75**(2):260-267. DOI: 10.1016/j.joms.2016.08.017

[38] Nitzan DW, Price A. The use of arthrocentesis for the treatment of osteoarthritic temporomandibular joints. Journal of Oral and Maxillofacial Surgery. 2001;**59**(10):1154-1160. DOI: 10.1053/joms.2001.26716

[39] Poluha RL, Canales GT, Costa YM, Grossmann E, Bonjardim LR, PCR C. Temporomandibular joint disc displacement with reduction: A review of mechanisms and clinical presentation [published correction appears]. Journal of Applied Oral Science. 2019;**27**:e2019er001. J Appl Oral Sci. 2019;27:e20180433. Published 2019 Feb 21. DOI: 10.1590/1678-7757-2018-0433

[40] Nitzan DW. The process of lubrication impairment and its involvement in temporomandibular joint disc displacement: A theoretical concept. Journal of Oral and Maxillofacial Surgery. 2001;**59**(1):36-45. DOI: 10.1053/joms.2001.19278

[41] Yoda T, Imai H, Shinjyo Y, Sakamoto I, Abe M, Enomoto S. Effect of arthrocentesis on TMJ disturbance of mouth closure with loud clicking: A preliminary study. Cranio. 2002;**20**(1):18-22. DOI: 10.1080/08869634.2002.11746185

[42] Polat ME, Yanik S. Efficiency of arthrocentesis treatment for different temporomandibular joint disorders. International Journal of Oral and Maxillofacial Surgery. 2020;**49**(5):621-627. DOI: 10.1016/j.ijom.2019.08.017

[43] Sanromán JF. Closed lock (MRI fixed disc): A comparison of arthrocentesis and arthroscopy. International Journal of Oral and Maxillofacial Surgery. 2004;**33**(4):344-348. DOI: 10.1016/j.ijom.2003.10.005

[44] Sanders B. Arthroscopic surgery of the temporomandibular joint: Treatment of internal derangement with persistent closed lock. Oral Surgery, Oral Medicine, and Oral Pathology. 1986;**62**(4):361-372. DOI: 10.1016/0030-4220(86)90282-3

[45] Nitzan DW, Samson B, Better H. Long-term outcome of arthrocentesis for sudden-onset, persistent, severe closed lock of the temporomandibular joint. Journal of Oral and Maxillofacial Surgery. 1997;**55**(2):151-158. DOI: 10.1016/s0278-2391(97)90233-0

[46] Nitzan DW, Marmary Y. The "anchored disc phenomenon": A proposed etiology for sudden-onset, severe, and persistent closed lock of the temporomandibular joint. Journal of Oral and Maxillofacial Surgery. 1997;**55**(8):797-803. DOI: 10.1016/s0278-2391(97)90335-9

[47] Stegenga B. Osteoarthritis of the temporomandibular joint organ and its relationship to disc displacement. Journal of Orofacial Pain. 2001;**15**(3):193-205

[48] Amir G, Goldfarb AW, Nyska M, Redlich M, Nyska A, Nitzan DW. 2-Butoxyethanol model of haemolysis and disseminated thrombosis in female rats: A preliminary study of the vascular mechanism of osteoarthritis in the temporomandibular joint. The British Journal of Oral and Maxillofacial Surgery. 2011;**49**(1):21-25. DOI: 10.1016/j.bjoms.2009.11.011

[49] Hoffman D, Puig L. Complications of TMJ surgery. Oral and Maxillofacial Surgery Clinics of North America. 2015;**27**(1):109-124

[50] Dohan DM, Choukroun J, Diss A, et al. Platelet-rich fibrin (PRF): A second-generation platelet concentrate.

Part I: Technological concepts and evolution. Oral Surgery, Oral Medicine, Oral Pathology, Oral Radiology, and Endodontics. 2006;**101**(3):e37-e44. DOI: 10.1016/j.tripleo.2005.07.008

[51] Dohan DM, Choukroun J, Diss A, et al. Platelet-rich fibrin (PRF): A second-generation platelet concentrate. Part II: Platelet-related biologic features. Oral Surgery, Oral Medicine, Oral Pathology, Oral Radiology, and Endodontics. 2006;**101**(3):e45-e50. DOI: 10.1016/j.tripleo.2005.07.009

[52] Wend S, Kubesch A, Orlowska A, et al. Reduction of the relative centrifugal force influences cell number and growth factor release within injectable PRF-based matrices. Journal of Materials Science. Materials in Medicine. 2017;**28**(12):188. Published 2017 Oct 25. DOI: 10.1007/s10856-017-5992-6

[53] Choukroun J, Ghanaati S. Reduction of relative centrifugation force within injectable platelet-rich-fibrin (PRF) concentrates advances patients' own inflammatory cells, platelets and growth factors: The first introduction to the low speed centrifugation concept. European Journal of Trauma and Emergency Surgery. 2018;**44**(1):87-95. DOI: 10.1007/s00068-017-0767-9

[54] Yuce E, Komerik N. Comparison of the efficiacy of intra-articular injection of liquid platelet-rich fibrin and hyaluronic acid after in conjunction with Arthrocentesis for the treatment of internal temporomandibular joint derangements. The Journal of Craniofacial Surgery. 2020;**31**(7):1870-1874. DOI: 10.1097/SCS.0000000000006545

[55] Albilia J, Herrera-Vizcaíno C, Weisleder H, Choukroun J, Ghanaati S. Liquid platelet-rich fibrin injections as a treatment adjunct for painful temporomandibular joints: Preliminary results. Cranio. 2020;**38**(5):292-304. DOI: 10.1080/08869634.2018.1516183

[56] Nazaroff J, Oyadomari S, Brown N, Wang D. Reporting in clinical studies on platelet-rich plasma therapy among all medical specialties: A systematic review of level I and II studies. PLoS One. 2021;**16**(4):e0250007. Published 2021 Apr 23. DOI: 10.1371/journal.pone.0250007

[57] Russo F, D'Este M, Vadalà G, et al. Platelet rich plasma and hyaluronic acid blend for the treatment of osteoarthritis: Rheological and biological evaluation. PLoS One. 2016;**11**(6):e0157048. Published 2016 Jun 16. DOI: 10.1371/journal.pone.0157048

[58] Pochini AC, Antonioli E, Bucci DZ, et al. Analysis of cytokine profile and growth factors in platelet-rich plasma obtained by open systems and commercial columns. einstein (Sao Paulo). 2016;**14**(3):391-397. DOI: 10.1590/S1679-45082016AO3548

[59] Lana JF, Weglein A, Sampson SE, et al. Randomized controlled trial comparing hyaluronic acid, platelet-rich plasma and the combination of both in the treatment of mild and moderate osteoarthritis of the knee. Journal of Stem Cells and Regenerative Medicine. 2016;**12**(2):69-78. Published 2016 Nov 29. DOI: 10.46582/jsrm.1202011

[60] Santagata M, De Luca R, Lo Giudice G, et al. Arthrocentesis and sodium hyaluronate infiltration in temporomandibular disorders treatment. Clinical and MRI evaluation. Journal of Functional Morphology and Kinesiology. 2020;**5**(1):18. Published 2020 Mar 6. DOI: 10.3390/jfmk5010018

[61] Chęciński M, Chęcińska K, Turosz N, Brzozowska A, Chlubek D, Sikora M. Current clinical research directions on

temporomandibular joint intra-articular injections: A mapping review. Journal of Clinical Medicine. 2023;**12**(14):4655. Published 2023 Jul 13. DOI: 10.3390/jcm12144655

[62] Israel HA, Diamond B, Saed-Nejad F, Ratcliffe A. Osteoarthritis and synovitis as major pathoses of the temporomandibular joint: Comparison of clinical diagnosis with arthroscopic morphology. Journal of Oral and Maxillofacial Surgery. 1998;**56**(9):1023-1028. DOI: 10.1016/s0278-2391(98)90246-4

[63] Afonso V, Champy R, Mitrovic D, Collin P, Lomri A. Reactive oxygen species and superoxide dismutases: Role in joint diseases. Joint, Bone, Spine. 2007;**74**(4):324-329. DOI: 10.1016/j.jbspin.2007.02.002

[64] Cristino S, Piacentini A, Manferdini C, et al. Expression of CXC chemokines and their receptors is modulated during chondrogenic differentiation of human mesenchymal stem cells grown in three-dimensional scaffold: Evidence in native cartilage. Tissue Engineering. Part A. 2008;**14**(1):97-105. DOI: 10.1089/ten.a.2007.0121

[65] Bonfante HL, Almeida CS, Abramo C, Grunewald STF, Levy RA, Teixeira HC. CCL2, CXCL8, CXCL9 and CXCL10 serum levels increase with age but are not altered by treatment with hydroxychloroquine in patients with osteoarthritis of the knees. International Journal of Rheumatic Diseases. 2017;**20**(12):1958-1964. DOI: 10.1111/1756-185X.12589

[66] Lou Y, Tao R, Weng X, Sun S, Yang Y, Ying B. Bioinformatics analysis of synovial fluid-derived mesenchymal stem cells in the temporomandibular joint stimulated with IL-1β. Cytotechnology. 2023;**75**(4):325-334. DOI: 10.1007/s10616-023-00579-x

[67] Wang T, He C. Pro-inflammatory cytokines: The link between obesity and osteoarthritis. Cytokine and Growth Factor Reviews. 2018;**44**:38-50. DOI: 10.1016/j.cytogfr.2018.10.002

[68] Kapoor M, Martel-Pelletier J, Lajeunesse D, Pelletier JP, Fahmi H. Role of proinflammatory cytokines in the pathophysiology of osteoarthritis. Nature Reviews Rheumatology. 2011;7(1):33-42. DOI: 10.1038/nrrheum.2010.196

Chapter 4

Operative Arthroscopy of the TMJ

Aly Mohamed Atteya

Abstract

TMJ arthroscopy is a minimally invasive procedure that has been used for treating internal derangement of the TMJ for years. It started with arthroscopic lysis and lavage and with time-operative procedures such as electrocoagulation, coblation, or even discopexy. It requires a high learning curve and a special instrument to be able to perform it. The instruments needed are usually delicate and can break easily such as the arthroscopic lens, the cannulas, the trocars and intraarticular instruments such as probe and scissors. It is done normally under general anesthesia, although few surgeons perform it locally. It gives very good results in most patients regarding improving mouth opening and pain reduction. Its complications are usually rare and can be avoided with excellent instrumentation and well-trained surgeons.

Keywords: TMJ, TMJ arthroscopy, minimally invasive, operative TMJ arthroscopy, temporomandibular joint, levels of TMJ arthroscopy, technique, complications

1. Introduction

Temporomandibular joint (TMJ) arthroscopy is a minimally invasive procedure that has been used for years for the treatment of internal derangement of the TMJ. The history of arthroscopy began in 1806 by Bozzini, who examined the intestinal bowel through an illuminated tube with a candle. Afterward, the first cystoscope was developed by Bruck in 1879. Using the cystoscope, Takagi made the first knee arthroscope in 1918. Eugene Bircher published the first scientific article on arthroscopy in 1921 [1].

Afterward, arthroscopy developed rapidly from 1960s to 1970s. The first arthroscope used in small joints was designed by Watanable in 1971. This instrument was 1.7 mm in diameter and could be inserted into a cannula of 2 mm. It had a light source, which provided better illumination, and a system called a "rod lens." It had a focal distance from 1 mm to infinity, which enabled the examination of small joints such as the elbow, wrist, and ankle. In 1973, O'Connor constructed an arthroscope with motorized elements for use during operations [2]. Ohnishi 1975 published the first article on diagnostic arthroscopy of the TMJ using the system that Watanable had described [3]. Hilsabeck and Laskin, in 1978, demonstrated that TMJ arthroscopy in rabbits was a safe technique to reveal the internal structures of the joint [4]. In 1982, the work on cadavers done by Murakami and Hoshinoi helped to define the regional arthroscopic anatomical nomenclature [5]. In 1983, McCain began a study on cadavers that included 67 joints, which helped in the description of the key anatomical points in order to make this technique safe and standardized [6]. On the other hand, studies began to appear with descriptions of the therapeutical benefits of TMJ arthroscopy in patients with acute or chronic closed lock, such as that of Sanders [7].

In 1986, Murakami and Ono described the elimination of intraarticular adhesions [8]. This was the starting point for the appearance of diverse arthroscopic techniques for treating different aspects and stages of temporomandibular disorders (TMDs). Professionals such as McCain, Sanders, Moses, Kolsin, Israel, Tarro and Yang developed sophisticated techniques for operative arthroscopy, including disc repositioning and suturing and the use of laser or radiofrequency [2].

2. Arthroscopy of the TMJ

We will discuss the different levels of TMJ arthroscopy, the instruments needed to perform the procedure, the arthroscopic anatomy inside the joint, the technique in detail, indications, results and complications.

2.1 Levels of TMJ arthroscopy

When we talk about the levels of TMJ arthroscopy, we are discussing different arthroscopic techniques, from the easiest and simplest one to the most difficult and complicated approach. There are three different levels of TMJ arthroscopy. Level I, which is a single puncture arthroscopy, has the same concept of arthrocentesis yet is done under vision using the arthroscope. It requires a learning curve from the surgeon to safely place a trocar with cannula in the superior joint space without causing damage to the joint or the adjacent structures such as the ear, brain or facial nerve. It allows diagnosis of the condition inside the joint, lysis and lavage of the inflammatory products, and the application of any therapeutic medications within the joint. It is the easiest technique of the three levels and requires less learning curve than the two other levels. Level II is done by double puncture and triangulation technique (will be explained later in the technique). It is an advanced technique and requires a higher learning curve from the surgeon. It enables the surgeons, in addition to the lysis and lavage done in level I, to perform intraoperative maneuvers inside the joint such as lateral pterygoid myotomy, electrocoagulation of the retrodiscal tissue, lysis of any adhesion, etc. Surgeons must perform many level I arthroscopy safely and perfectly before upgrading their technique to level II. Level III is the most difficult and sophisticated technique; it requires much more higher learning curve and is done by double puncture and triangulation technique and triple punctures in certain techniques. It is the same as level II, but at the end of the procedure, discopexy is done. There are many techniques of arthroscopic discopexy like the McCain suturing technique [9], Yang suturing technique [10], and the technique of Martin-Granizo using the resorbable pin for disc fixation [11]. Usually, these techniques necessitate a customized special instrument that is not produced regularly in the market yet done especially for them.

2.2 Instruments of TMJ arthroscopy

The quality and availability of the instruments needed for TMJ arthroscopy are very important in the success of the procedure. Bad quality of the instruments or lack of some important instruments may affect the success of the procedure. We will discuss the different types of instruments needed to perform the procedure.

- Arthroscopic lens. It varies in diameter and angulation; usually, the accepted diameter to use inside the joint ranges from 1.9 to 2.7 mm and the length from 40 to 70 mm. The angulation can be 0 degrees or 30 degrees. Different companies manufacture this lens. It should be handled cautiously by the surgical team as it can be broken easily.

- Cannulas for the lens and for the instruments. The number of cannulas needed depends on the technique. It ranges from one to three cannulas. Their diameter ranges from 1.5 to 3 mm.

- Sharp and blunt trocars are to be used with the cannulas.

- Light source with a light cable will be connected to the cannula.

- Video cameras, which are many types, from the standard definition to the full high definition (FHD) and 4 K, it is better to be connected to a computer to record video and images during the procedure.

- Endoscopic monitor or television screen.

- Intraarticular instruments such as palpator, scissor, grasper, scalpel.

- Source of energy to be used inside the joint such as laser and radiofrequency such as the coblator.

We will describe now in detail the main instruments needed for the arthroscopy.

2.2.1 The arthroscopic lens

The lens system consists of an objective lens, which must be positioned close to the object needed to be viewed, and an eyepiece that should be close to the viewer's eye in case the surgeon wants to view the surgical field directly through the lens or can be connected to a camera and transmit the view into a monitor. The lens has a rod, which is usually 5 cm long and is connected to the camera by either a system of clips or threads (**Figure 1**). They usually have a diameter between 1.9 and 2.7 mm. The rod lens of Hopkins represents the evolution of the small diameter endoscope. It improves the transmission of light and expands the field of vision. The optical part should be handled with extreme care during the operation and afterward during washing and sterilization as it is very delicate and can be broken easily. Each lens has a field of vision, which is the angle formed from the tip of the arthroscope to the lateral edges of the field. It is 60 degrees in most types of the lens (that range from 1.9 to 2.7 mm in diameter). Some companies have a wider field of vision of 80 degrees, and usually, they are more expensive. The lens is divided into two types according to its angle of inclination, 0 degrees and 30 degrees. The inclination angle is the angle formed between a line that passes through the center of the field of vision of the lens and a line that passes through the long axis of the lens. The 0-degree arthroscope (**Figure 2**) is not suitable for level II or level III but is satisfactory for level I arthroscopy because it can only give a vision of the area situated in front of it as its end is not beveled (**Figure 3**). This will result in some angles inside the joint not being visible because the space inside the joint is very tiny, and you cannot move the arthroscope freely inside it. The 30-degree arthroscope (**Figure 4**) is excellent for level II and level III and of course

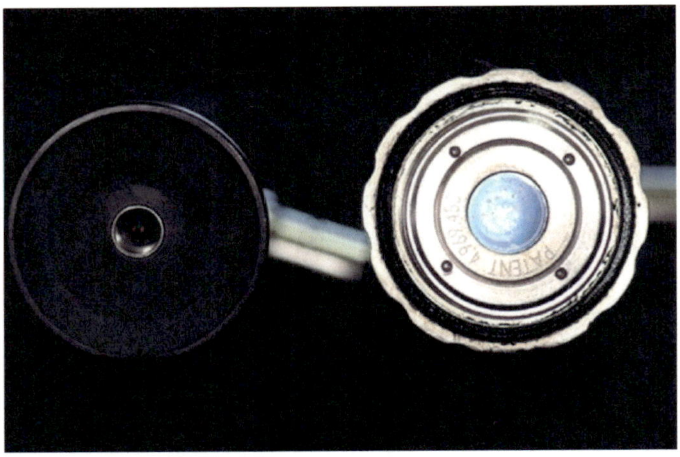

Figure 1.
Clips system for connection with the camera on the left and threads system on the right (photo courtesy of Prof. Florencio Monje Gil) [2].

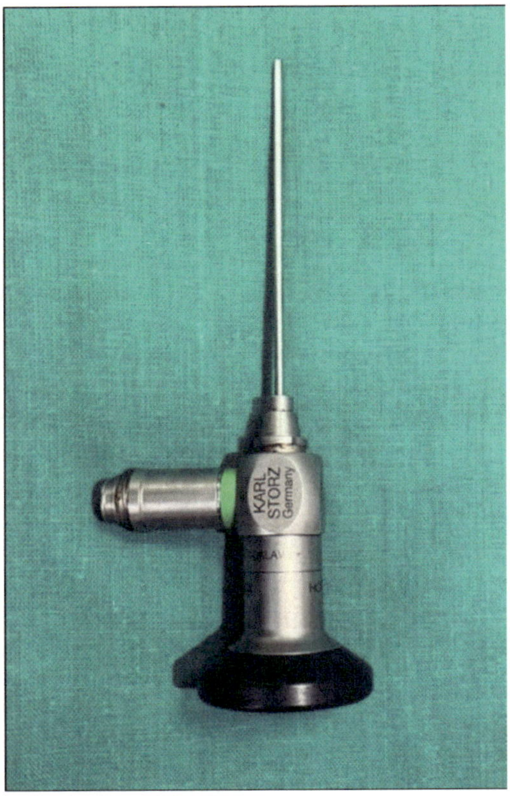

Figure 2.
The 1.9 mm 0-degree arthroscopic lens.

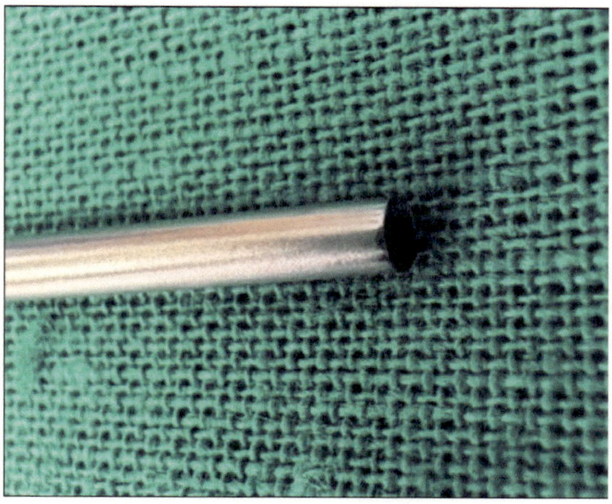

Figure 3.
The end of the 0-degree arthroscopic lens shows no bevel.

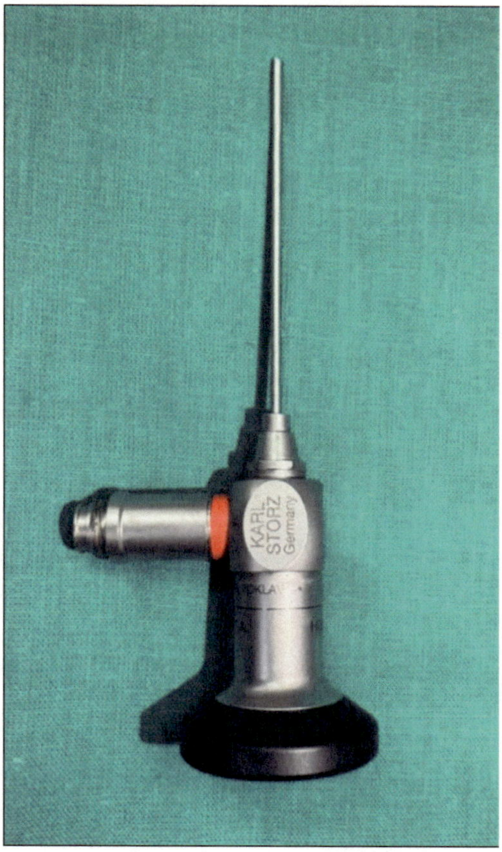

Figure 4.
The 1.9 mm 30 degrees arthroscopic lens.

can be used in level I. It can give a view of all angles inside the joint without the need to exert huge and excessive movements inside this small joint. This happens by rotating the arthroscope around its axis, and with every turn, it gives a view of a different angle. For example, if the 30-degree bevel (**Figure 5**) is facing downward (this is the neutral position), it gives a view of the area in front and below it. If we rotate the arthroscope and the bevel is facing to the right side, it gives a view to the area on the right side; if it is facing upwards, it gives a view to the area situated upward from the scope, etc. We can notice that this happens without moving the arthroscope, only rotating around its long axis. This is very important to allow the surgeon to do the triangulation technique (which will be explained later in the technique) and view his second cannula.

2.2.2 Cannulas and obturators

The cannulas (**Figures 6** and **7**) are the tubes into which the arthroscopic lens and the surgical instruments are inserted. They are at least 0.1 mm larger than the diameter of the arthroscope, which permits the entry of solution inside the joint. They have marks on their shafts indicating the length every 5 mm, and thus, they can indicate the depth inside the joint. Some of them have an entry port, others two or even a spigot, to allow injection of any solution inside the joint. The obturators (**Figures 8** and **9**) are pen-shaped tools that allow the cannula to penetrate inside the joint for the initial placement.

2.2.3 Light source and light cable

The light source is the source that delivers light needed for illumination inside the joint to allow better visualization of the joint cavity by the surgeon. It is either halogen or xenon. The xenon is better as it emits more natural and brighter light. The light cable (**Figure 10**) transmits the light from the light source to the arthroscopic lens to illuminate the joint.

2.2.4 Video camera

At the beginning of the arthroscopy, surgeons performed the operation by looking directly through the lens of the arthroscope without any camera or monitor.

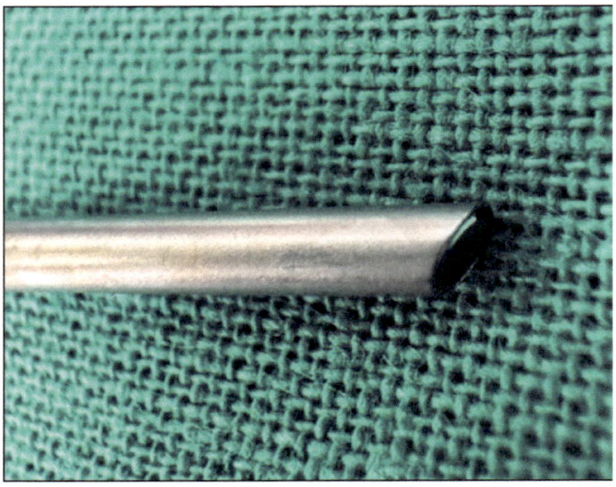

Figure 5.
The end of the 30-degree arthroscopic lens with the bevel.

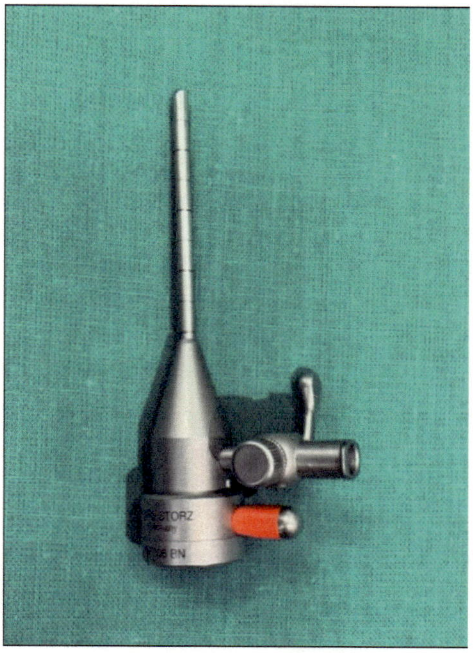

Figure 6.
Cannula for the 30-degree arthroscopic lens. It is marked every 5 mm and has a spigot for the entry of solutions.

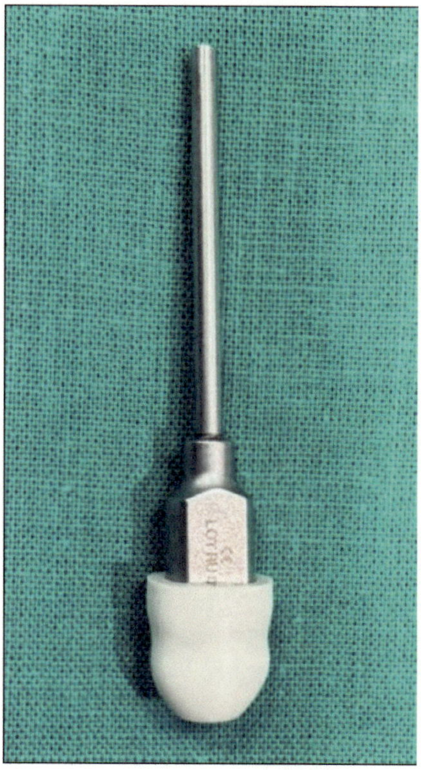

Figure 7.
Cannula without any entry port for the solutions, used only for the entry of instruments inside the joint.

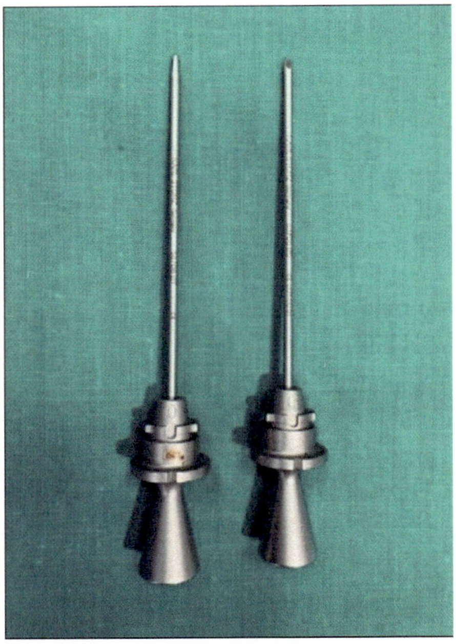

Figure 8.
Sharp (on the right) and blunt (on the left) obturators, to be used with the cannula of the lens.

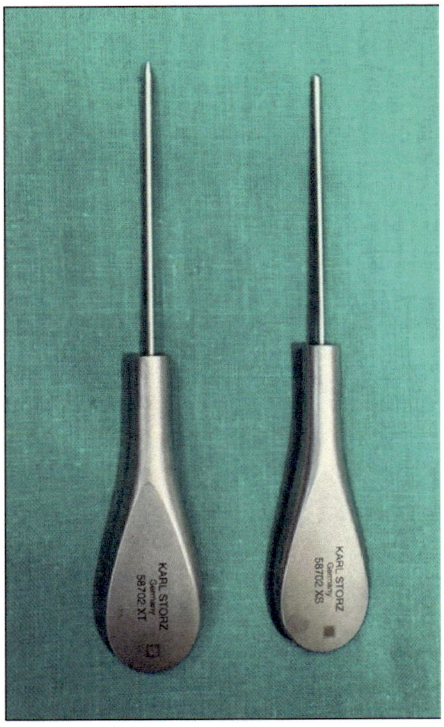

Figure 9.
Sharp (on the right) and blunt (on the left) obturators, to be used with the small cannula of instruments.

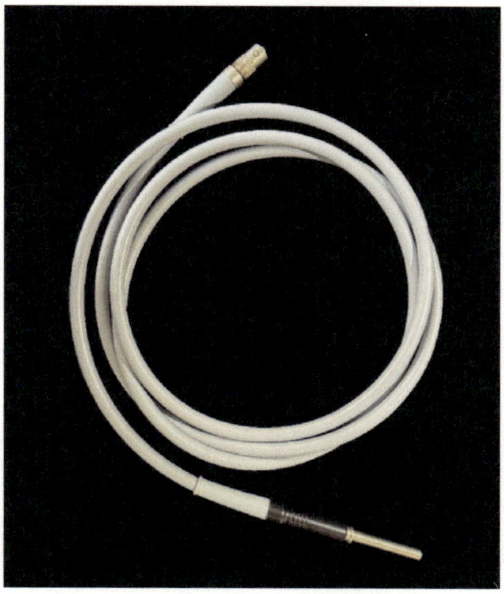

Figure 10.
The light cable.

Subsequently, after the development of video cameras and monitors, it becomes possible to use this technology in the medical field. With the help of small video cameras, which are connected to the arthroscopic lens and connected at the same time with a central console where the image is processed, an image was successfully viewed on a monitor, and this allowed all the members of the surgical team and even the trainee to watch the operation. The video of the operation and images can be recorded for educational use eventually or for restudy of the case with the surgical team if needed. The system consists of two parts: (a) the video camera (**Figure 11**), which can be HD,

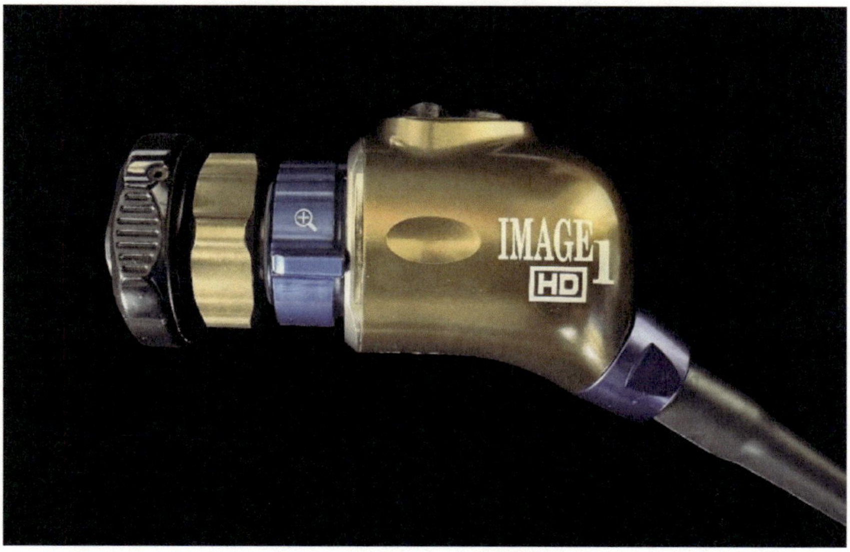

Figure 11.
The video camera. The blue arm is for adjusting the zoom, and in front of it is a gold arm for adjusting the focus.

FHD, 4 K, or even 3D. It is connected to the arthroscopic lens. It has a multifunction button that can be customized for special functions such as zoom, recording, taking images, etc. (b) The central console (**Figure 12**) where the image is processed to be shown on the monitor.

2.2.5 Endoscopic monitor

It is a special screen on which the video of the operation is presented (**Figure 13**). Normal TV screens can also be used. These screens have developed from the old heavy and thick tubes to the current slim and high-definition monitors. They vary in size and definition, from the HD to the FHD and now the 4 and 8 K.

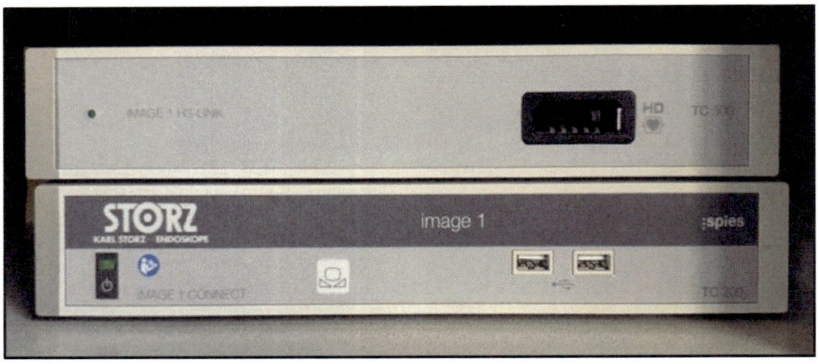

Figure 12.
The central console.

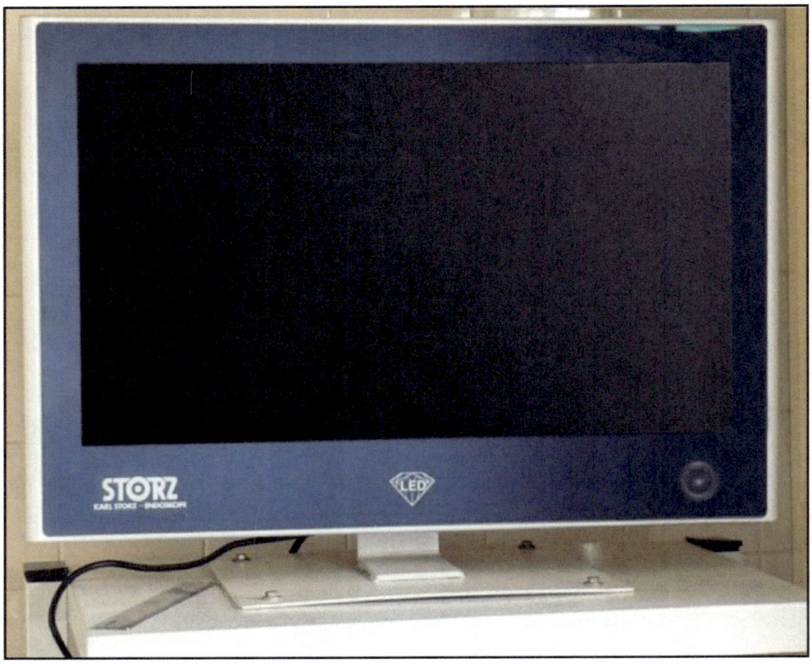

Figure 13.
The endoscopic monitor.

2.2.6 Intraarticular instruments

These are small instruments used for the operative procedure inside the joint. Their size allows them to enter inside the joint through the small-sized sheath. They are palpators, graspers, scissors, and scalpel.

The palpator (**Figure 14**) is an instrument that allows the surgeon to palpate any surface inside the joint, detach any adhesions, and try to mobilize the disc. It can be angled or straight. The angled palpator is ideal for palpating the articular eminence and thus detecting the presence of chondromalacia and its degree. It is better and safer than the straight one as it can induce perforation and iatrogenic injury in the weakened area inside the joint such as the disc.

The grasper (**Figure 15**) is used to extract anything inside the joint, such as blood clots, pathological tissue for biopsy, and any foreign body. It can be straight, curved or scissor type.

The scissor (**Figure 16**) is used to cut any adhesions, open the capsule, or even cut part of the muscle. It has a type with a fixed upper jaw and moving lower jaw and another type with the opposite, with a fixed lower jaw and moving upper jaw.

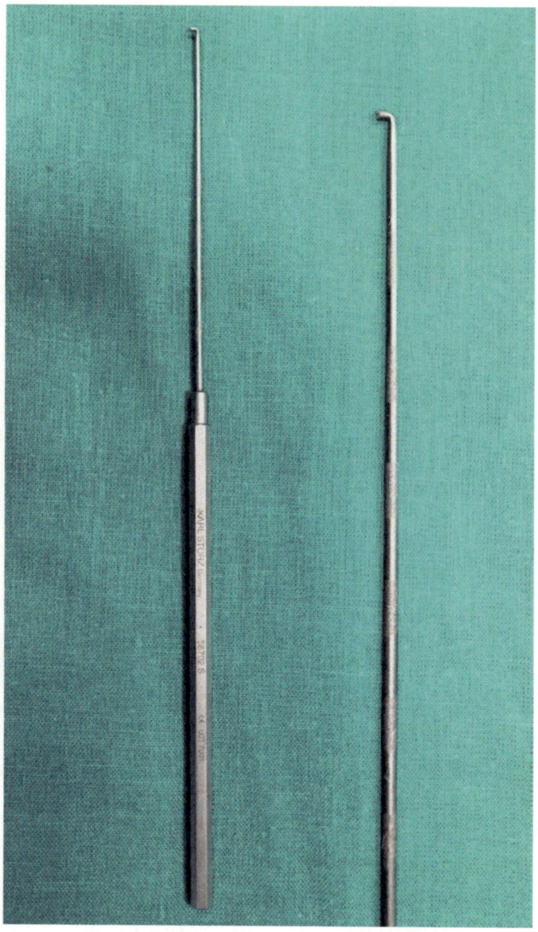

Figure 14.
The palpator on the left and the right a magnification of its tip.

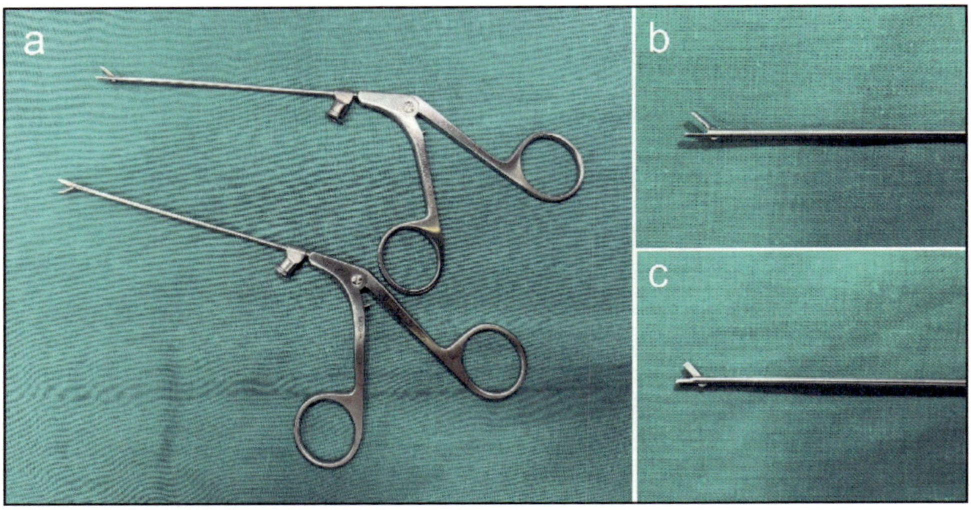

Figure 15.
(a) Two different types of graspers: above is the straight one and below is the scissor type, (b) is a magnification of the straight one and (c) is the scissor one.

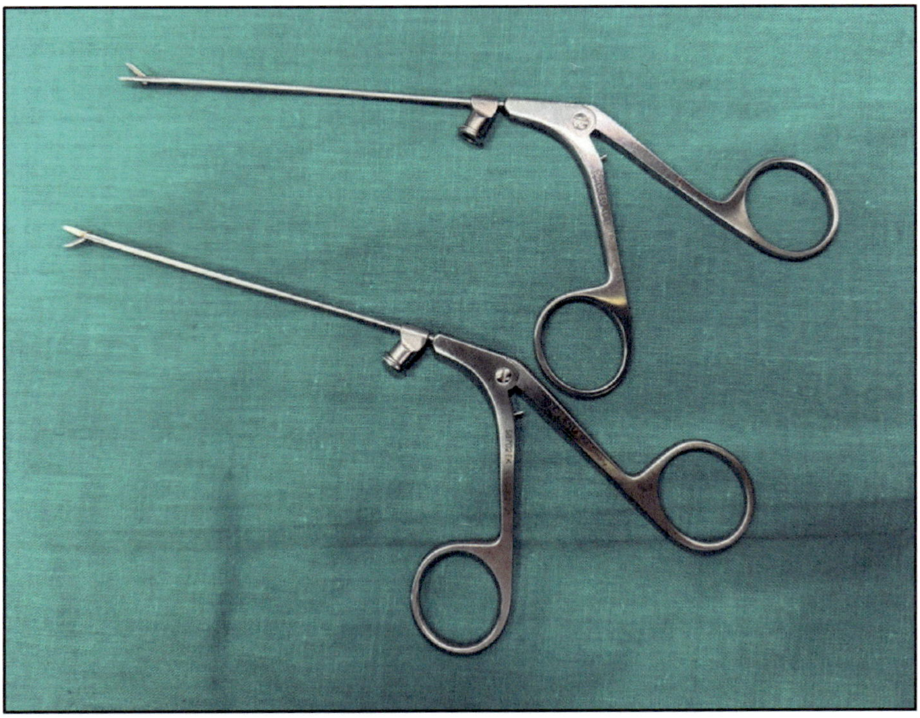

Figure 16.
Two different scissors; the one above has a moving upper jaw and the one below has a moving lower jaw.

The scalpel (**Figure 17**) is also used for cutting but mainly for the anterior bands. It has different shapes according to the tip. It should be used cautiously inside the joint as it can cause iatrogenic injury and hemorrhage.

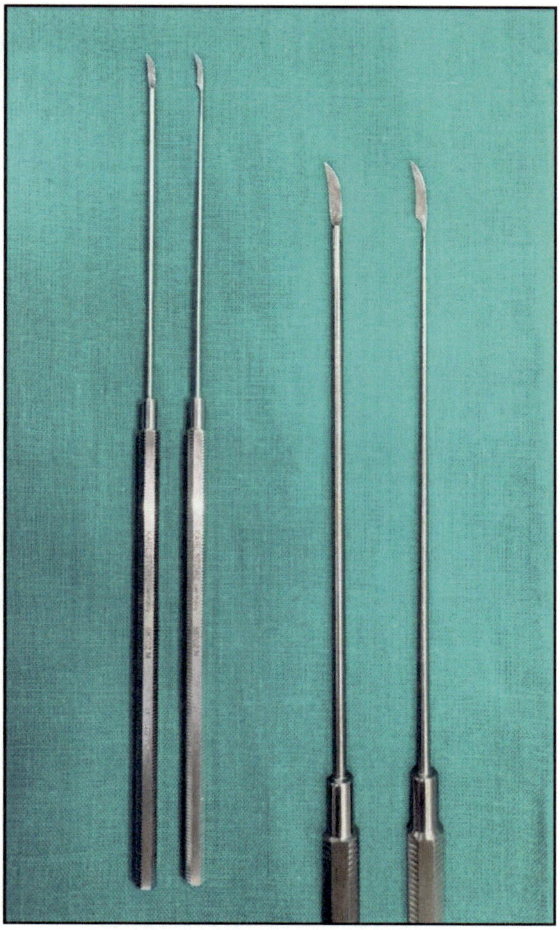

Figure 17.
Two different scalpels.

2.2.7 Source of energy to be used inside the joint

Many sources of energy can be used inside the joint such as the monopolar diathermy, the laser and the radiofrequency. The monopolar diathermy is not the preferred source inside the joint as it generates more heat inside the joint that could be lethal to the chondrocyte and produce fumes that can affect the quality of image of the arthroscopic lens if used many times and with time, the picture becomes unclear. The laser can be used inside the TMJ as a source of energy. The ND-Yag laser is the most used type.

Radiofrequency is a type of energy that denaturalizes and destroys the protein of the cell, or in other terms, it evaporates the cell. It is more precise than the monopolar diathermy and produces less heat. The most famous one is the coblator (**Figure 18**) of Smith and Nephew, which is widely used in otorhinolaryngology. It is used for evaporation of any synovitis inside the joint, myotomy of the muscle and electrocoagulation of the retrodiscal tissue. The type of handle used for the coblator is the flex 45 degrees handle (**Figure 19**), which was originally used by otorhinolaryngology to treat turbinate hypertrophy.

Figure 20 shows how the devices are arranged on the arthroscopic tower.

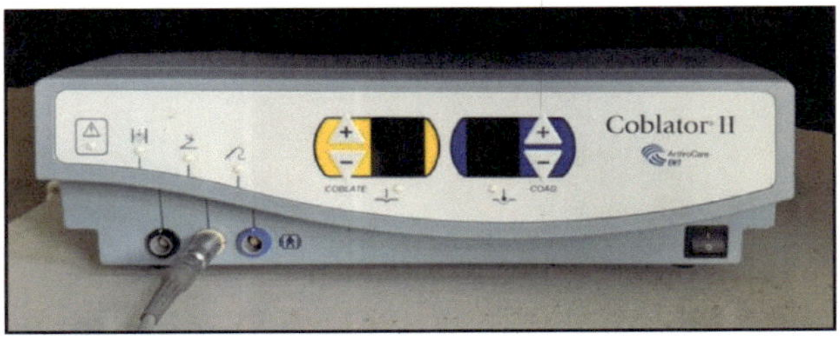

Figure 18.
Coblator II of Smith and Nephew.

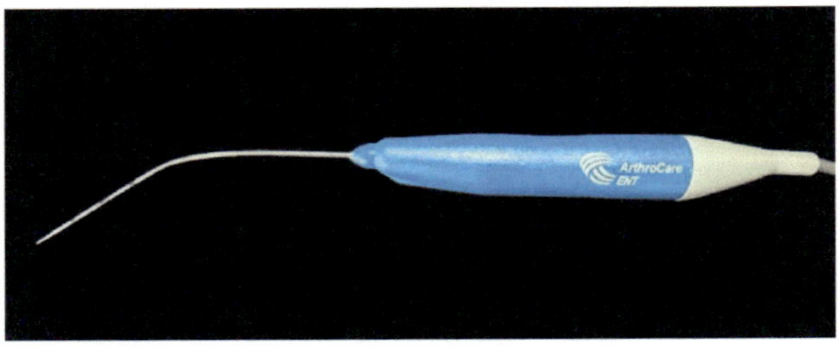

Figure 19.
The flex 45-degree handle of the coblator. Usually, it is unbent before being used in TMJ arthroscopy.

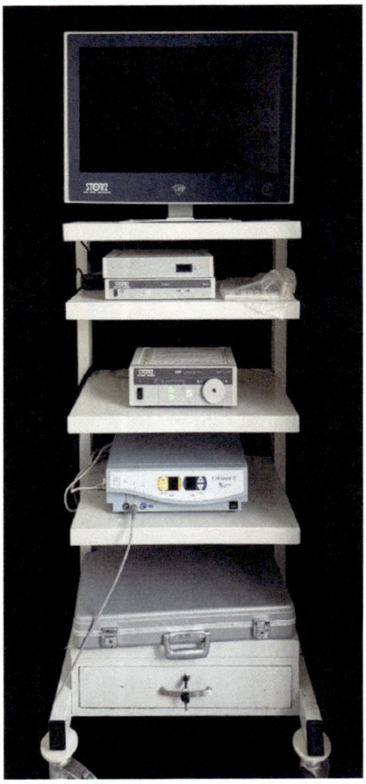

Figure 20.
The arthroscopic tower.

2.3 Important anatomical landmarks

It is important to know the main anatomical landmarks inside the joint before doing any procedure. Usually, the procedure is done in the superior joint space, so when we talk about important anatomical landmarks, we mean the superior joint space. As a rule, the joint should be inspected from the inside outwards and from back to front. It is also advisable to move from known places to unknown places. If, at some point, we are incapable of locating an area or features, we can return to the starting point. The articular eminence is a very important landmark to be considered. Anytime we get lost inside the joint, we should return to it; thus, it will be easy to recognize the anatomy again. There are seven areas (**Figure 21**) to be examined in the superior joint space [12]:

1. Medial synovial drape

2. Pterygoid shadow

3. Retrodiscal synovium:

4. Posterior slope of articular eminence and glenoid fossa

5. Articular disc

6. Intermediate zone

7. Anterior recess

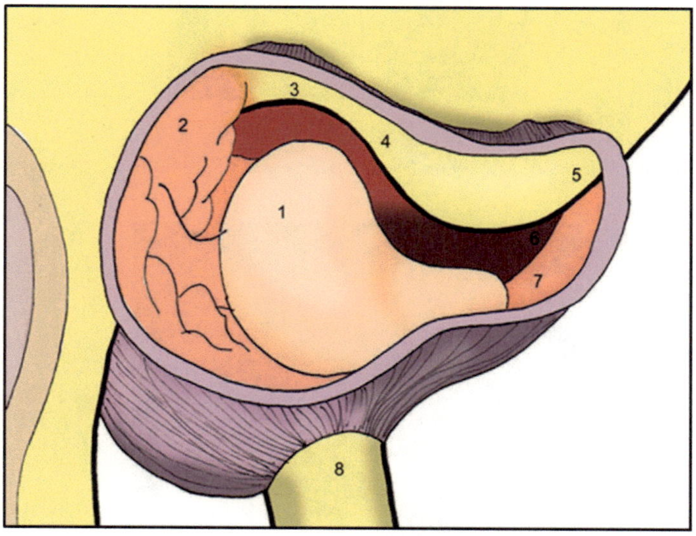

Figure 21.
The seven areas to be examined in the superior joint space. (1) articular disc, (2) synovial lining in the posterior recess, (3) glenoid fossa, (4) posterior slope of the eminence, (5) articular eminence, (6) medial part of the anterior recess where the pterygoid shadow can be seen, (7) lateral part of the anterior recess, eight condyle (photo courtesy of Dr. Raúl Gonzalez Garcia) [12].

1. Medial synovial drape: (**Figures 22–24**) It is the first anatomic landmark and the first area to be examined at the beginning of arthroscopy. Normally, it is a grayish-whitish area with minimal capillary proliferation that is seen in the tissue. It has striae that run up and down a tissue and a tense appearance. At acute inflammatory stages, it becomes more reddish instead of grayish-white, and the proliferation of capillaries, hyperemia, and petechias are seen.

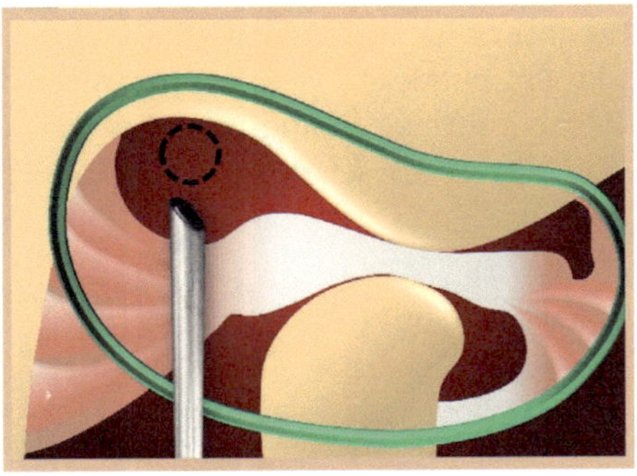

Figure 22.
Diagram shows the position of the arthroscope and aspect of the medial synovium.

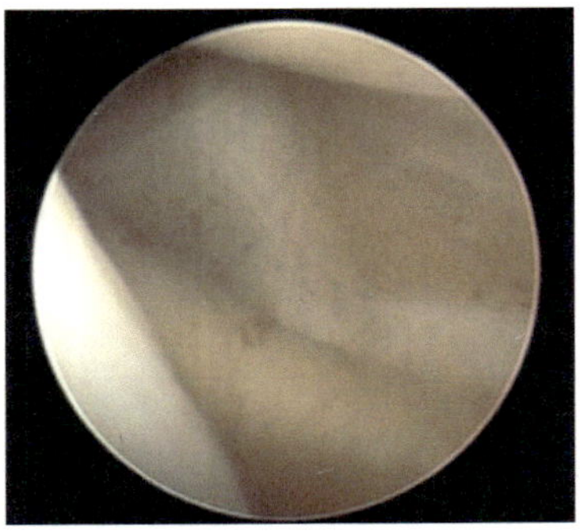

Figure 23.
Arthroscopic view of a healthy medial synovium (photo courtesy of Dr. Raúl Gonzalez Garcia) [12].

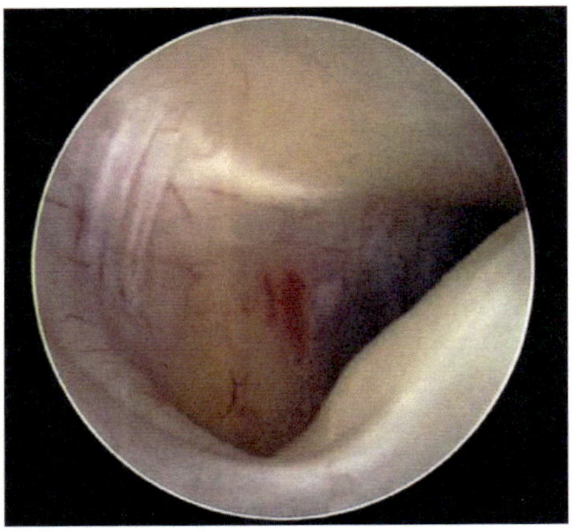

Figure 24.
Arthroscopic view of a hyperemic medial synovium (photo courtesy of Dr. Raúl Gonzalez Garcia) [12].

2. Pterygoid window (**Figures 25–27**): It is an area present in the medial synovium anterior to the medial synovial drape. Usually, it is purple in color, which is the reflection of the pterygoid muscle under the synovial lining. In pathological stages, it can be hyperemic with hypervascularization and even perforation and herniation of the muscle.

3. Retrodiscal synovium: (**Figures 28–30**) It is a smooth and thin tissue rich in blood vessels and nerve endings. This area can be reached by moving the arthroscope laterally and posteriorly. It can be divided into three zones:

   a. Oblique protuberance, which is in the middle third of the retrodiscal synovium. It is the posterior attachment of the disc that is covered with synovial lining. When the condyle moves during the opening of the mouth, it becomes more prominent and appears as a crest or crease.

   b. Retrodiscal tissue is inserted in the posterior part of the glenoid fossa.

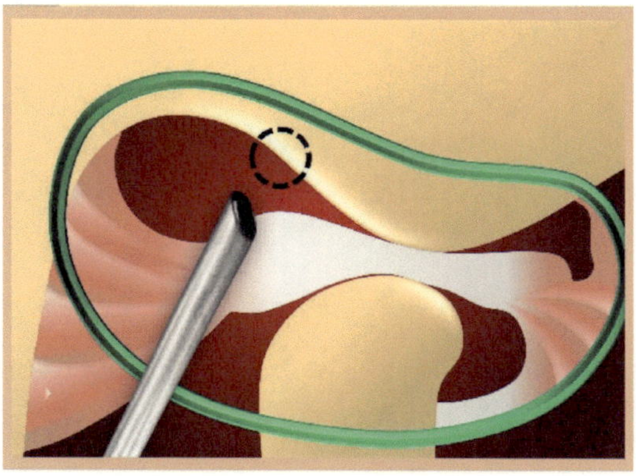

Figure 25.
Diagram shows the position of the arthroscope and the appearance of a pterygoid shadow.

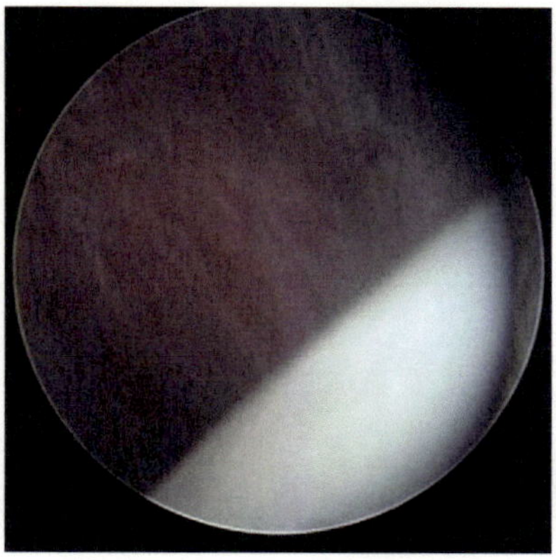

Figure 26.
Arthroscopic view of a healthy pterygoid window (photo courtesy of Dr. Raúl Gonzalez Garcia) [12].

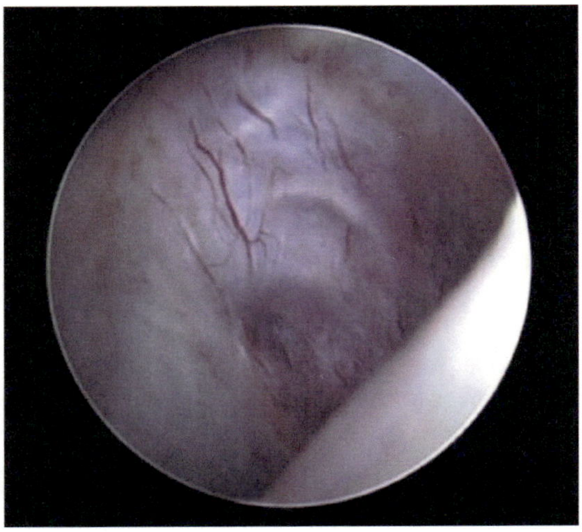

Figure 27.
Arthroscopic view of a hyperemic pterygoid window (photo courtesy of Dr. Raúl Gonzalez Garcia) [12].

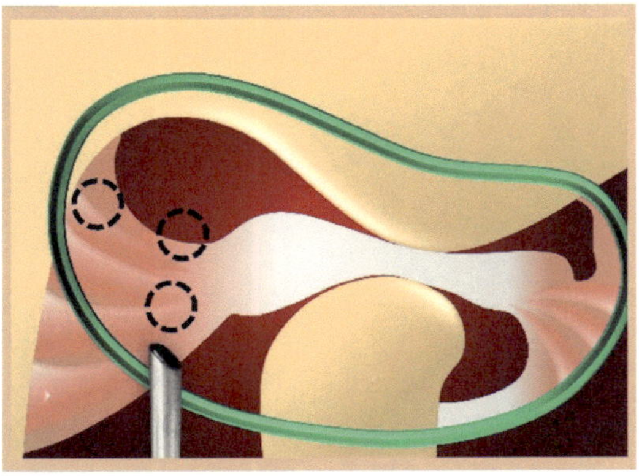

Figure 28.
Diagram shows the appearance of retrodiscal synovium.

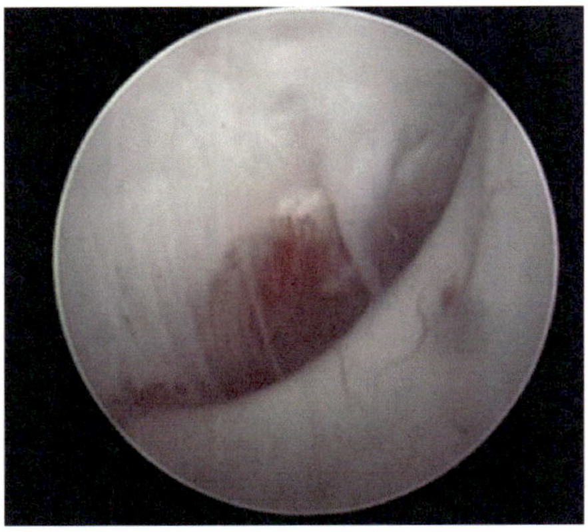

Figure 29.
Arthroscopic view of a healthy retrodiscal synovium (photo courtesy of Dr. Raúl Gonzalez Garcia) [12].

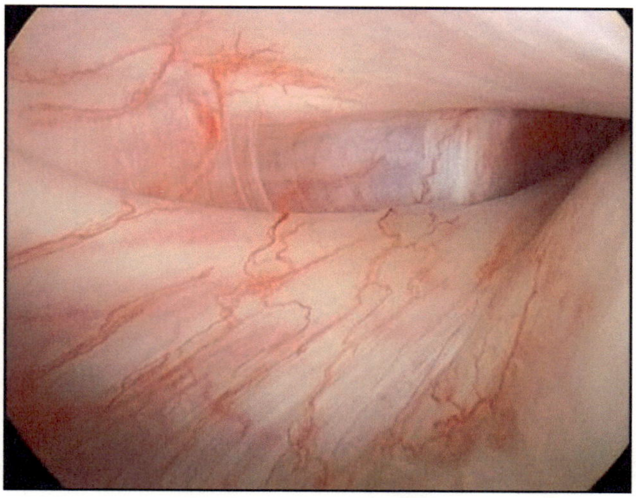

Figure 30.
Arthroscopic view of a hyperemic retrodiscal synovium (photo courtesy of Prof. Florencio Monje Gil) [2].

c. Lateral recess of the retrodiscal synovial tissue. It is the most lateral part of the synovial tissue and can be seen by moving the arthroscope laterally. This zone appears tense and is rich in capillaries. In pathological cases, this area appears reddish due to hyperemia.

4. Posterior slope of the articular eminence and glenoid fossa: (**Figures 31** and **32**) When the arthroscope is directed toward the most medial portion of the posterior slope, the fibrocartilage appears white with anteroposterior striae. By moving the arthroscope backward toward the glenoid fossa, it becomes darker and thinner. When the fibrocartilage becomes pathologically thin, the underlying bone appears slightly yellowish, and this is known as chondromalacia.

5. Articular disc: (**Figures 33** and **34**) Normally, it is white in color with a smooth surface, without irregularities or depressions. The disc is avascular structure, and the capillaries of the retrodiscal synovium will end where the posterior portion of

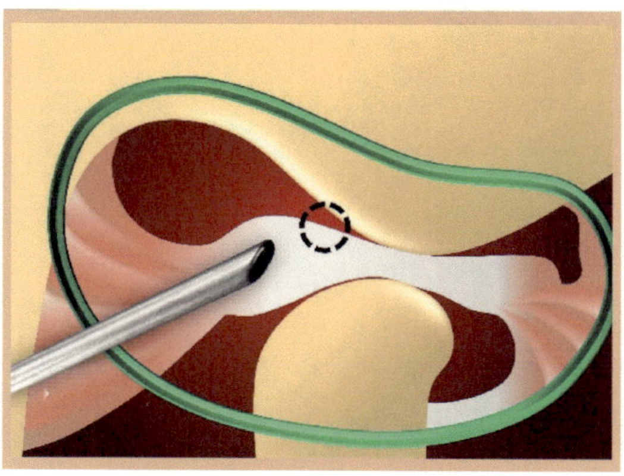

Figure 31.
Diagram shows the posterior crest of the articular eminence.

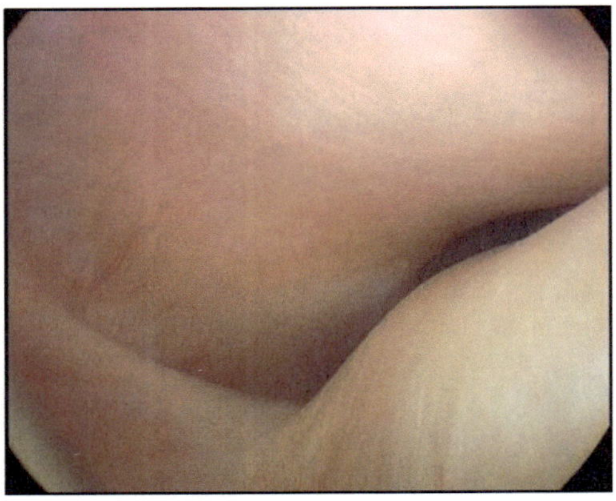

Figure 32.
Arthroscopic view of the posterior crest of the articular eminence (photo courtesy of Prof. Florencio Monje Gil) [2].

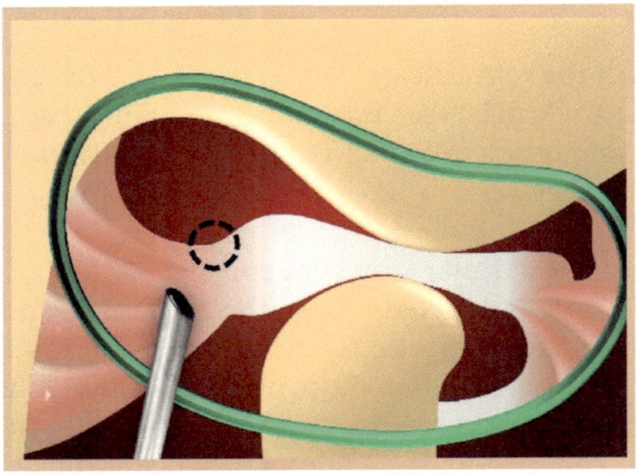

Figure 33.
Diagram shows the appearance of articular disc (photo courtesy of Prof. Florencio Monje Gil) [2].

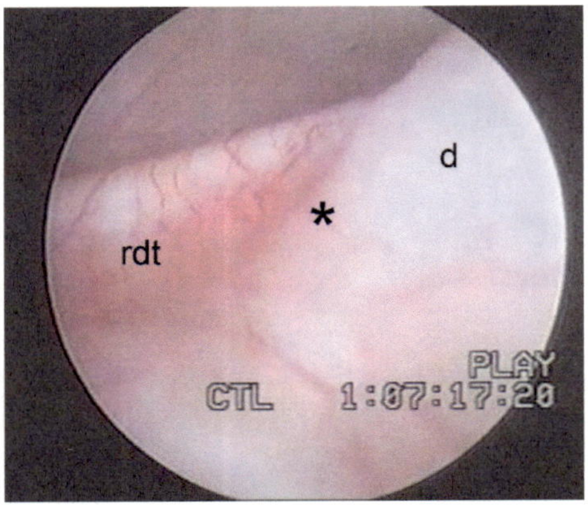

Figure 34.
*Arthroscopic view showing the retrodiscal tissues rdt, the joint disc d, and the interface between the two structures * (photo courtesy of Prof. Florencio Monje Gil) [2].*

the disc begins. The junction between the retrodiscal synovium and the posterior band of the disc form normally has a U-shaped depression, which can disappear or be a more acute depression in case of disc displacement. Disc mobility is tested by putting the arthroscope in a lateral position and asking the assistant to open and protrude the patient's mandible; naturally, the disc glides over the articular eminence without problems. One important concept when evaluating the position of the disc is the degree of roofing, which evaluates the percentage of the articular disc that covers the condyle. Roofing is graded arthroscopically according to the posterior band of the articular disc in relation to the articular eminence. When the mouth is opened (the condyle is in a forward position), roofing is considered 100% if the posterior band of the disc is lying adjacent to the posterior slope of the articular eminence. This happens when the disc is in a normal position. When the mouth is closed (the condyle is seated), roofing is 100% if the posterior band of the disc is present approximately at the midportion of the glenoid fossa.

6. Intermediate zone: (**Figures 35** and **36**) It is the zone between the anterior and posterior recess; when the arthroscope is directed toward it, we usually see the anterior surface of the articular eminence, the disc inferiorly, and the synovium of the anterior recess. It has significance in determining the position of the disc and, thus, the degree of roofing. When the disc is normal in position, it is white on white (the white color of the anterior slope is on the white color of the disc). In case of anterior disc displacement, it is white (the white color of the anterior slope) on red (the red color of the retrodiscal synovium).

7. Anterior recess: (**Figures 37** and **38**) To be able to reach the anterior recess, we ask the assistant to close the mandible of the patient in order to bring the condyle within the temporal fossa, and we move the arthroscope laterally and anteriorly until the anterior synovium is identified. This recess is relatively difficult to reach, especially if the articular eminence is steep. It is the place where the second cannula should be placed.

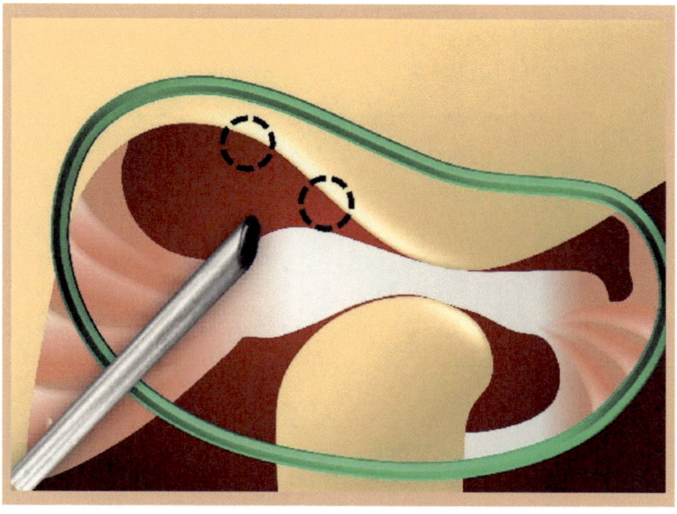

Figure 35.
Diagram shows aspect of the intermediate area (photo courtesy of Prof. Florencio Monje Gil) [2].

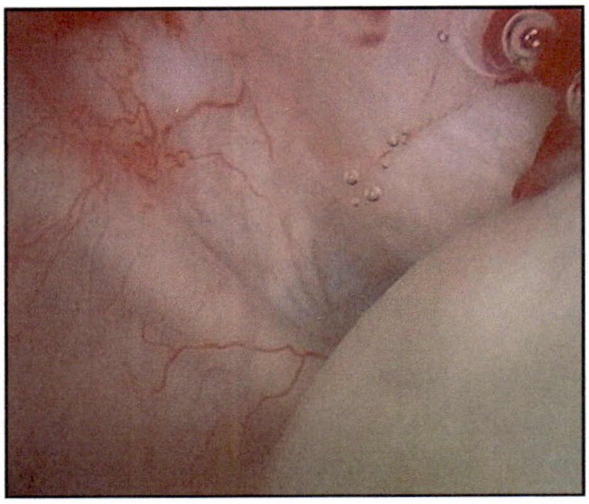

Figure 36.
Arthroscopic view showing the intermediate area (photo courtesy of Prof. Florencio Monje Gil) [2].

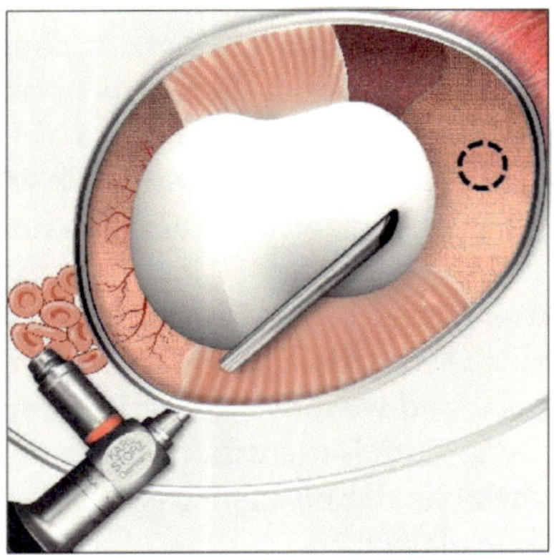

Figure 37.
Diagram shows the anterior recess.

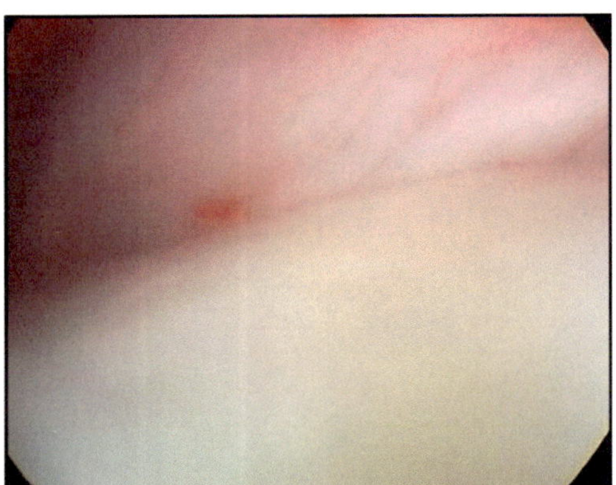

Figure 38.
Arthroscopic view of the anterior recess (photo courtesy of Prof. Florencio Monje Gil) [2].

2.4 Technique

The procedure is usually done under general anesthesia. Some surgeons perform it under local anesthesia, especially level I arthroscopy, and very few surgeons perform level II or III under local anesthesia.

1. The patient's head is positioned in a supine position and then turned gently to the contralateral side to place the head in a lateral position (**Figure 39**). In some patients, the preauricular area is shaved or we can paint the hair with gel and then put adhesive bandages on the temporal area to prevent falling of hair in the surgical field. A cotton or gauze is put in the patient's ear and then the patient is painted with betadine. Afterwards, sterile drapes are placed in a manner that allows the surgical assistant to place his fingers in the patient's oral cavity.

2. The position of the surgeon, staff and surgical material is shown in **Figure 40**

3. With a sterile marker, we draw the Holmlund and Hellsing line, which is a line between the tragus of the ear and the outer canthus. On this line, a point that is 10 mm in front of the tragus and 2 mm under is usually the site of the first entry, which coincides with the maximum concavity of the glenoid fossa. Before putting the first needle inside the joint, the joint is felt by the nailing method (**Figure 41**). This is done by asking the assistant to open the mouth and pull the mandible forward; a depression can be felt, and this will be the site where the first needle will be put. An intramuscular needle is inserted at this point in the medial direction, back to front and below to above, until we touch bone (the glenoid fossa), and this is a sign that we are inside the joint (**Figure 42**). It aims to inject intraarticular solution to distend the joint and allow ease of insertion of the first puncture.

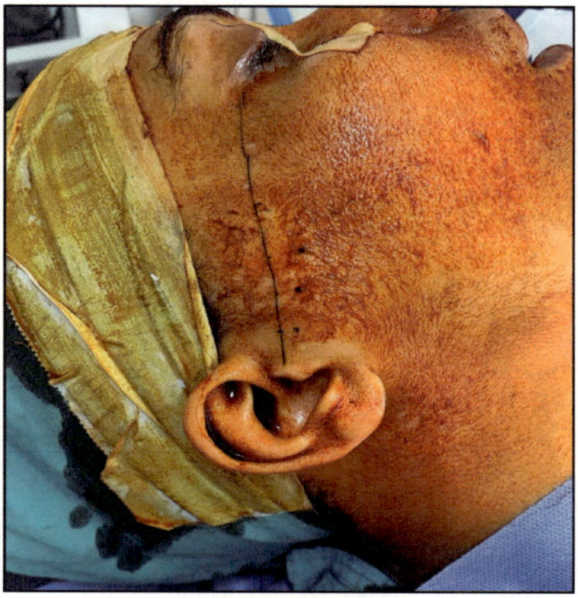

Figure 39.
Placement of adhesive bandage and sterile drapes to delineate and isolate the surgical field.

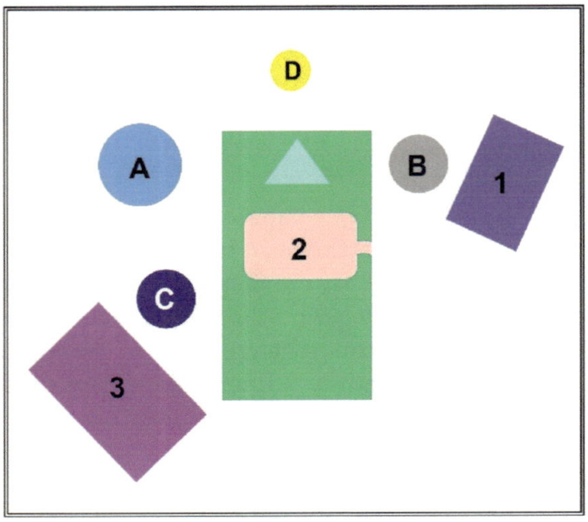

Figure 40.
(A) Surgeon. (B) Surgical assistant. (C) Nursing staff. (D) Arthroscope tower. (1) Anesthesia table. (2) The main basic sterilized instruments. (3) Surgical table with complementary sterilized instruments.

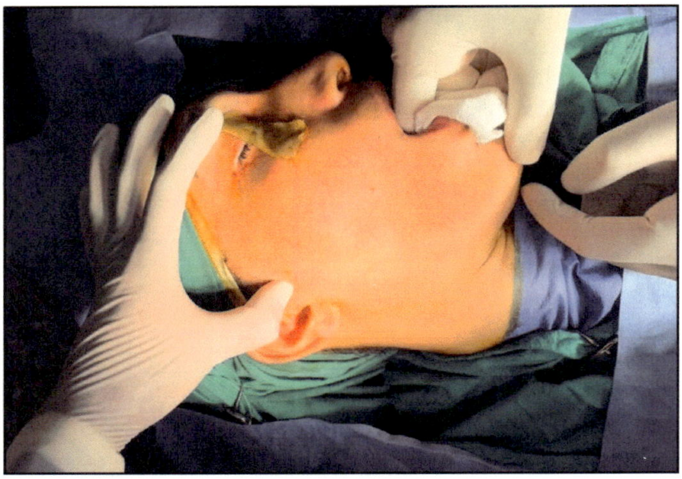

Figure 41.
Nailing method to palpate the joint.

4. The needle was removed gently, and then a cannula with a sharp trocar was inserted inside the joint with the help of rotating movement in the same direction used to insert the needle. This should be done with the assistant pulling the mandible downward and forward. We continue advancing the trocar until it touches the bone of the zygomatic arch just above the glenoid fossa (**Figure 43**). At this point, we use the sharp trocar as a dissector to open the joint capsule and enter the superior joint space by gentle movement. When the sensation of entering the joint is felt, the sharp trocar is changed to the blunt one to avoid undue damage to the joint surfaces. The blunt trocar is then removed, and the arthroscope is ready to be inserted (**Figure 44**).

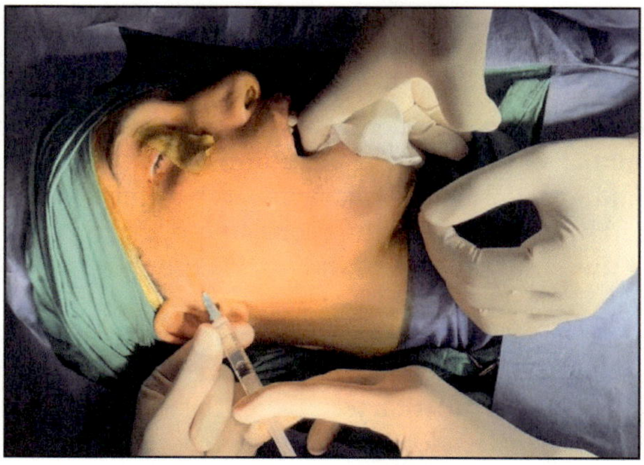

Figure 42.
Intramuscular needle injection of the superior joint space with the aid of assistant who is pulling the mandible downwards and forwards.

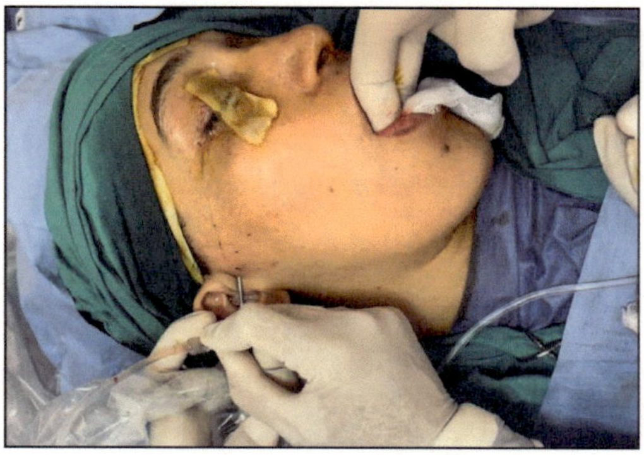

Figure 43.
Insertion of the first cannula.

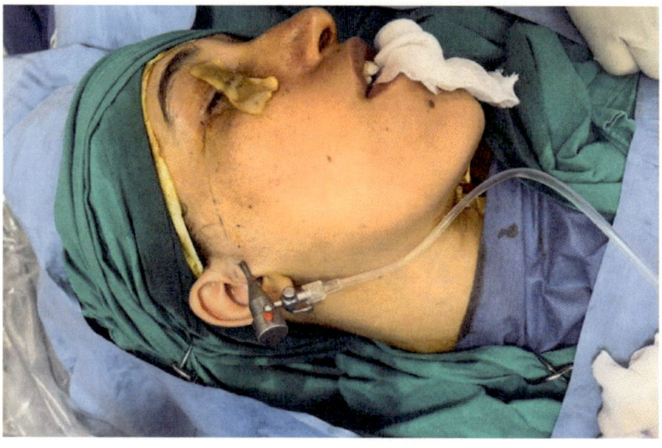

Figure 44.
After insertion of the first cannula.

5. The arthroscope is then inserted into the cannula (**Figures 45** and **46**) and fixed to it by a key-hole mechanism. The joint is irrigated with a ringer lactate solution to distend it and maintain clear vision. Normal saline solution is not preferred as it is hyperosmolar and could be lethal to chondrocytes. After that, a needle was inserted in front and below the first puncture, which serves as a drainage port (**Figures 47** and **48**). We begin exploration of the joint at the seven areas previously discussed by moving the arthroscope anteroposterior and mediolateral and by rotation of the lens if 30 degrees was used (**Figures 49** and **50**).

6. The second cannula will be inserted at the anterior recess under direct arthroscopic visualization. This step is tricky and requires a high learning curve. It is inserted using the triangulation technique. The idea of triangulation is making an equilateral triangle that allows the surgeon to visualize the second cannula inside the joint. For example, if the depth of the first cannula inside the joint is 25 mm, we take a point away from it by 25 mm and then insert the second cannula perpendicular at a depth of 25 mm (**Figure 51**). To insert the second cannula, the arthroscope is moved as far anteriorly and laterally as possible from the articular eminence. The depth of the first cannula was recorded when the arthroscope was placed at that position. The second cannula was inserted perpendicularly at a point located at an equal distance to the depth of the first cannula (**Figures 52–54**). The thirty-degree lens is very useful in this step as it can be

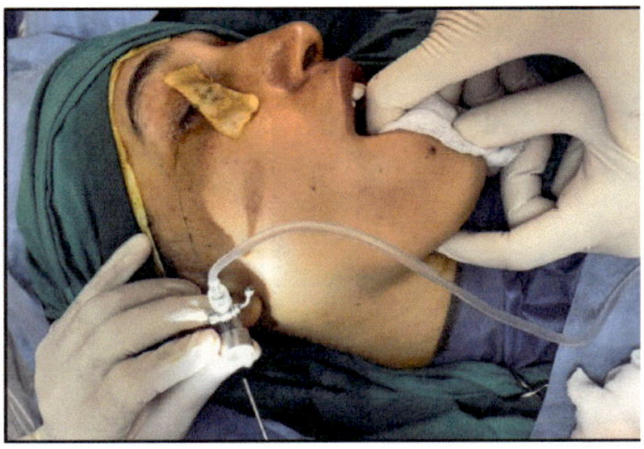

Figure 45.
During insertion of the arthroscope inside the sheath.

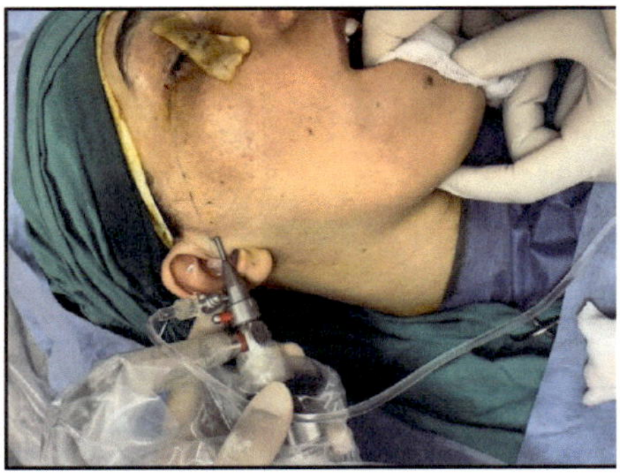

Figure 46.
The arthroscope is inserted into the sheath.

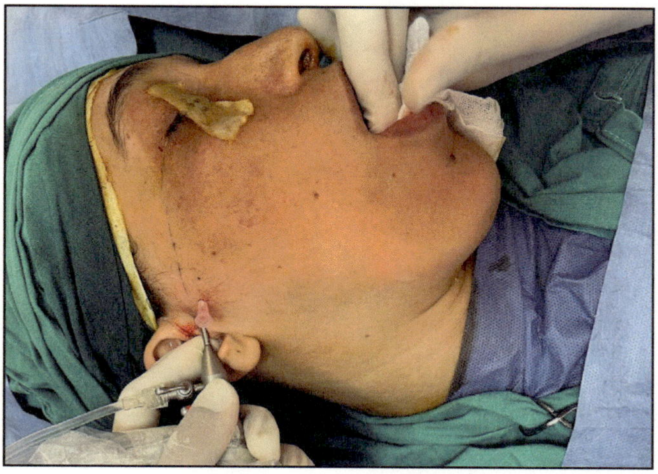

Figure 47.
The is inserted as a drainage port.

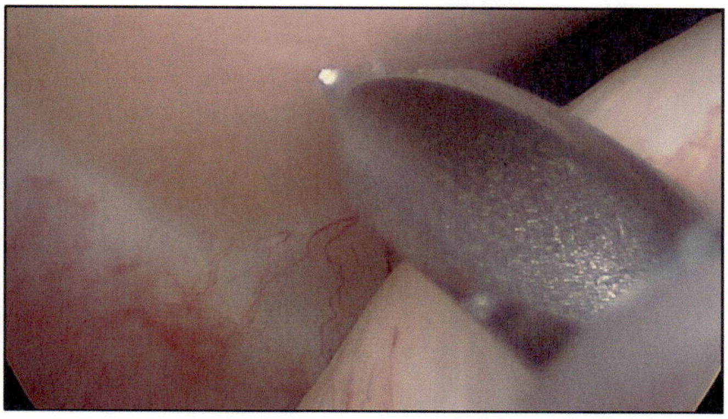

Figure 48.
View of the needle inside the joint.

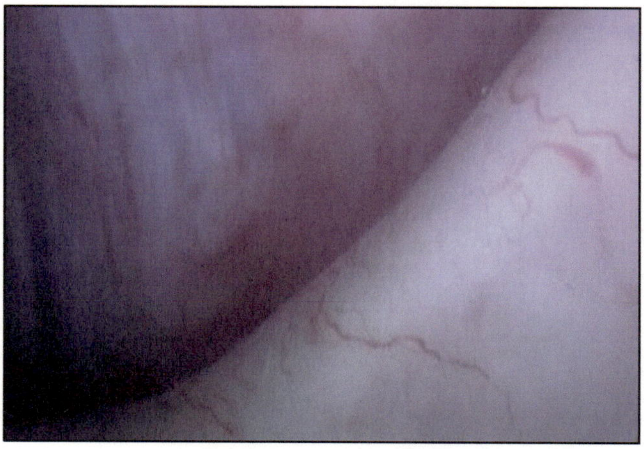

Figure 49.
Posterior recess showing the retrodiscal tissue.

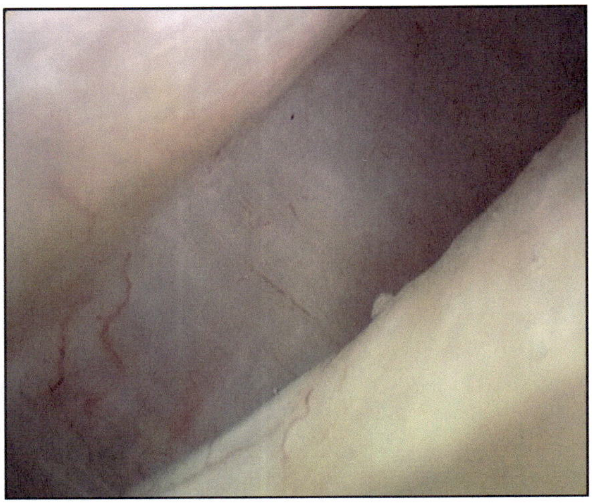

Figure 50.
Anterior recess showing the lateral pterygoid shadow.

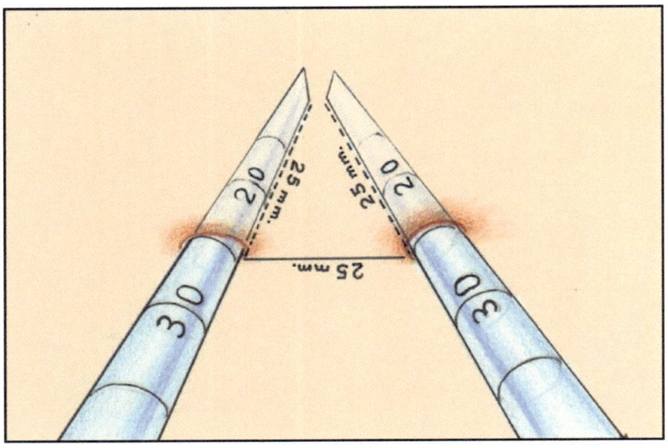

Figure 51.
Schematic drawing explains the triangulation technique (photo courtesy of Prof. Florencio Monje Gil) [2].

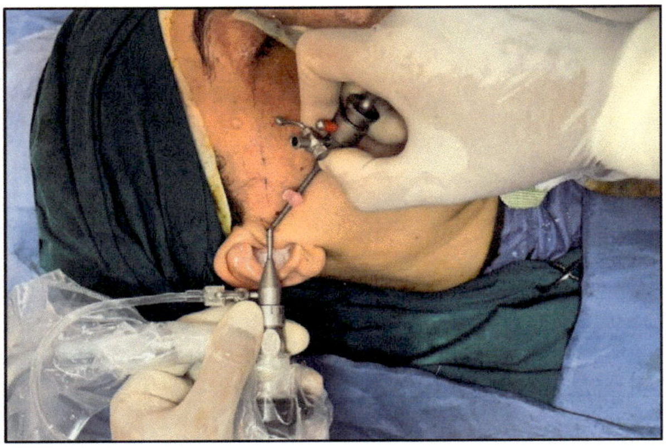

Figure 52.
Measurement of the distance to insert the second cannula (it is inserted away from the first cannula at the same distance of its depth).

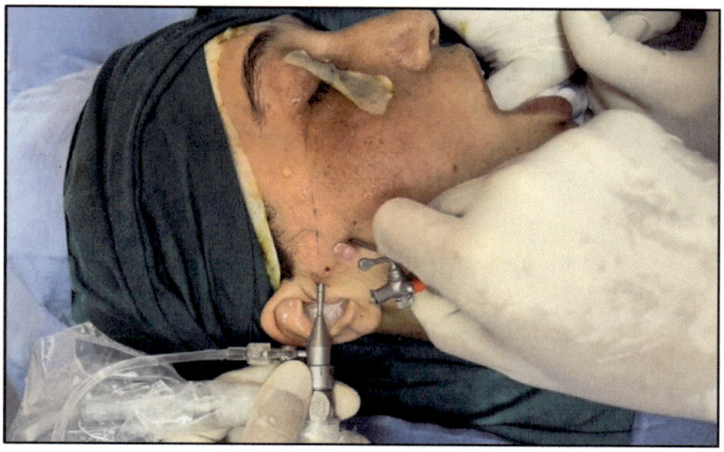

Figure 53.
Insertion of the second cannula.

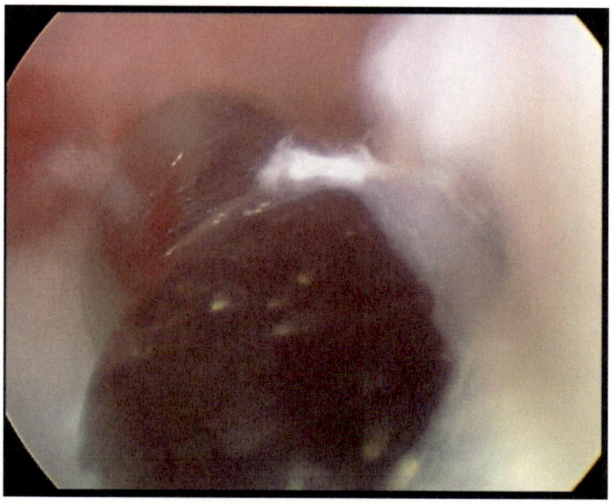

Figure 54.
View of the entry of second cannula inside the joint.

rotated 360 degrees in all directions to give different angles of vision. In this way, an equilateral triangle is formed between the two cannulas.

7. Through the second cannula, we can insert small instruments. We begin inserting the coblator (**Figure 55**) to release any adhesion and do a myotomy in the lateral pterygoid muscle to cut the anterior attachment of the disc with the muscle. The incision line is located approximately 2–3 mm anterior to the anterior band of the disc and is carried out across the whole width from medial to lateral. The depth of the anterior release should not be more than 2–4 mm to avoid bleeding from large blood vessels and injuring the masticatory muscle nerve in the anteromedial synovium (**Figures 56** and **57**). After the release, electrocoagulation of the retrodiscal tissue with the coblator (**Figure 58**) is done, aiming to coblate the nerve endings responsible for the pain and inducing fibrosis that helps the

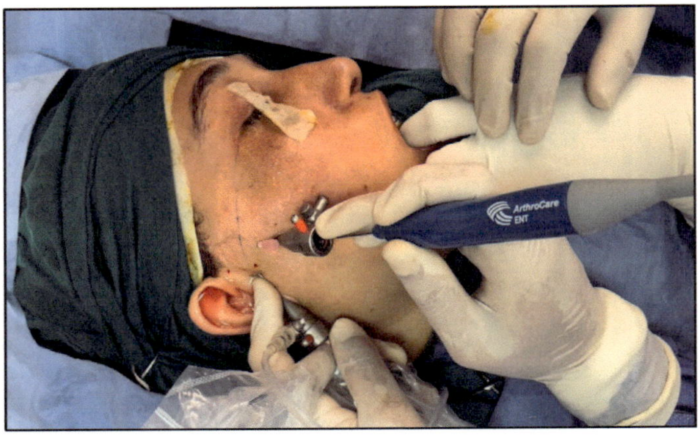

Figure 55.
The introduction of the coblator to be used inside the joint.

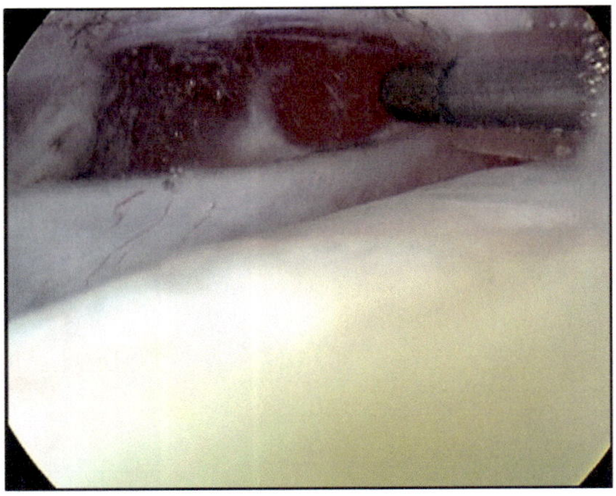

Figure 56.
The beginning of lateral pterygoid myotomy using the coblator.

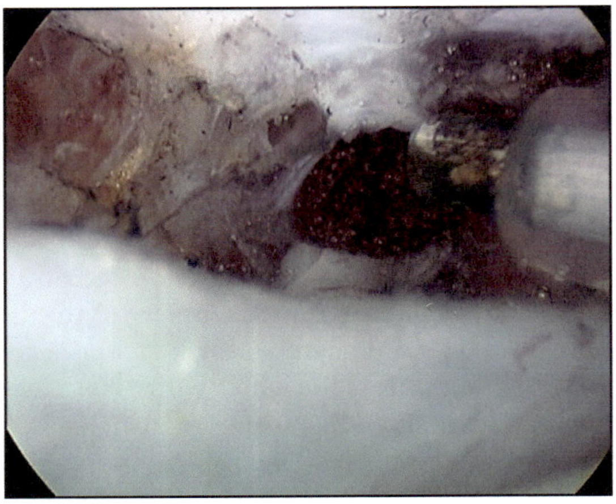

Figure 57.
Almost finishing the myotomy at the desired depth.

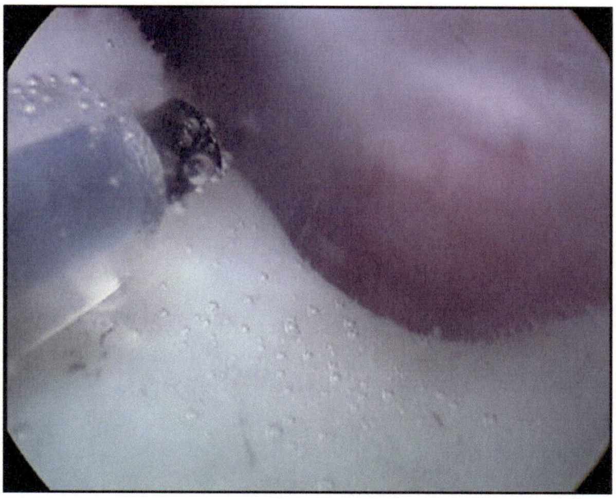

Figure 58.
Electrocoagulation of the retrodiscal tissue.

anteriorly displaced disc to return to its normal position. In the end, coblation of any synovitis or inflammation in the joint should be done.

8. At the end of the procedure, the obturator of the disc is pushed backward by any blunt instrument. Immediately after, the second cannula is removed, and we can inject some medication inside the joint such as sodium hyaluronate or PRP through the first cannula after removal of the arthroscope.

9. If level III arthroscopy is done either by suturing or resorbable pins, it is done before injecting the medication. For further reading about level III, read the papers of Joseph McCain [9], Chi Yang [10] and Martin-Granizo [11].

2.5 Postoperative management

Antibiotics and nonsteroidal anti-inflammatory drugs are routinely prescribed for 3 days. A soft diet is advised for 2 months and is decreased gradually. Any food that needs a knife to be cut should be avoided, and any food that can be cut with a fork should be eaten instead. Exercises to improve mouth opening were explained to the patient and started 1 week after the operation.

In patients with significant postoperative occlusal changes, a splint was recommended. It was designed to raise the bite and prevent contact between upper and lower incisors and canines. Due to the resulting distalization of the bite force, joint loading was reduced, which contributed to the joint's rehabilitation. The appliance was left in place around the clock during the first ten postoperative days and then used at night for four additional weeks.

2.6 Indications and contraindications

TMJ arthroscopy has now become the treatment of choice for TMJ internal derangement after failed conservative treatment. Despite this, it is not suitable for treating all the pathologies of the TMJ. The American Association of Oral and Maxillofacial Surgery stated five indications:

- Internal derangement with pain and dysfunction.
- Wilkes stage II, III and IV.
- Synovitis.
- Hypermobility with painful joint or recurrent jaw dislocation.
- Hypomobility because of intraarticular adhesions.
- Degenerative joint diseases which have the lowest success rate.

Holmlund et al. [13], and Sanders et al. [14], have argued for additional indications:

- TMJ arthropathy due to systemic arthritis.
- TMJ problems following orthognathic surgery.
- Biopsy.
- When there is no relation between clinical and radiological findings.

There are some contraindications of the TMJ arthroscopy:

- Previous open TMJ surgery.
- Suspicions of tumor.
- Cutaneous, ear or joint infection.
- Fibrous or bony ankylosis.
- Patient with steep articular eminence (it is a relative contraindication, especially for level II and III, as it will be difficult to access the anterior recess and insertion of the second port).

2.7 Results

The main goal for the management of any TMJ pathology is to reduce pain, reestablish normal mandibular movements and improve the quality of life for patients. Many treatment modalities have been reported to treat internal derangement of the TMJ such as conservative treatment (muscle relaxants, anti-inflammatory, etc.), arthrocentesis, TMJ arthroscopy and open joint surgery. Currently, there is no consensus regarding the most effective treatment for patients with internal derangement of TMJ. There are many clinical studies that have investigated the efficacy of various treatment modalities for the management of internal derangement. However, the best treatment modality with predictable outcomes based on solid evidence is still unclear. [15] Sanders in 1986 was the first author to show the beneficial effect of TMJ arthroscopy. He found that it was a successful technique for cases with acute or chronic locked jaw. [7] Nitzan and Dolwick found a 70% improvement in the symptoms of patients who were treated with arthroscopic lysis and lavage. [16] Indresano investigated TMJ arthroscopy on 64 patients with a follow up from 9 to 30 months. [17] He considered three parameters: reduction of pain postoperatively, mouth opening, and the need for further treatment after the procedure. Improvement was noted in 73% of the patients, and the best results were achieved in patients with acute or chronic locking, with 83% improvements. Montgomery [18] conducted a study of arthroscopic lysis and lavage in 19 patients with a follow up 6–12 months. He showed a 90% improvement; however, 50% of the patients had residual pain. In 1989, Moses et al. [19] conducted a study on 152 joints with disc displacement without reduction, in which they used a blunt and pointed trocar for lysis of adhesion. They suggest making anteroposterior movements with the cannula. 92% of the patients showed a decrease in pain and 78% had a maximum mouth opening of 40 mm. Moses and Poker [20], in the same year, studied TMJ arthroscopy on 237 patients, with an average follow-up of 19 months. They found that 92% of the patients had decreased pain and increased mouth opening. They discovered that a bad prognosis was associated with cases that had condylar osteophyte. Israel and Roser [21] found improvement in pain and mouth opening after arthroscopic lysis and lavage in 25 joins with an average follow-up of 7.5 months. In 1991, Clark et al. [22] found that 57% of the patients had a decrease in pain intensity after TMJ arthroscopy and an 83% increase in mouth opening. The same research group conducted a study in 1993 [23] on patients with joint locking. The results were analyzed with 2 years follow-up. They found significant improvement in patients regarding pain and mouth opening. They concluded that disc position has little impact on the symptoms of the patients since they improved after lysis and lavage, and the procedure did not affect the disc position. Machon and Hirjak et al. [24] conducted a study about arthroscopic lysis and lavage on 50 patients with chronic anterior disc displacement without reduction. They divided the patients into two groups according to the chronicity of symptoms: group A (patients with symptoms less than 1 year) and group B (patients with symptoms more than 1 year). They found that inflammatory changes in retrodiscal tissue and synovium were 71% in group A and 82% in group B, while fibrous adhesion was present in 14% of group A and 45% in group B, and degenerative changes of the disc and articular surface were present in 4% of group A and 32% in group B. They found a significant increase in mouth opening and pain reduction in both groups but more in group A. They concluded that patients benefit from arthroscopic lysis and lavage, but patients with shorter duration of symptoms benefit more. Ahmed and Sidebottom [25] reported in their study that arthrocentesis and arthroscopy have significant improvement in 86% of patients who had previously taken conservative treatment and did not improve, and the best results were in patients with Wilkes stage II and III. Murakami [26] made a study of the outcome of TMJ arthroscopy with 5-year follow-ups. He had a success rate that ranged from 86% in Wilkes III to a surprising 93% at Wilkes V. He recommended advanced arthroscopic surgery (laser, discoplasty, synovectomy) at stage V. Moses and Topper [27] have used MRI in patients who were treated with arthroscopic lysis and lavage. It was effective in 90% of the patients, although the MRI shows that the disc continues in anterior displacement position in 92% of the patients. They concluded that the success of lysis and lavage is not due to disc repositioning but probably linked to disc mobilization, elimination of inflammatory products, and denervation of the capsule as a result of the surgical procedure. All these factors will help joint adaptation, regeneration and remodeling. However, Chi Yang et al. [28] in their study showed the importance of disc position in TMJ arthroscopy. They found new bone formation in the previously diseased mandibular condyle over time when the disc is repositioned over the condyle (arthroscopic discopexy using level III arthroscopy). González-Garcia et al. [29] had a study with 458 patients (611 joints) with internal derangement of TMJ from Wilkes II to IV. They compared arthroscopic lysis and lavage with operative arthroscopy in a 2-year follow-up period. Both groups had a significant decrease in pain without significant differences between the two groups. The highest decrease in pain and increase in mouth opening was in patients with Wilkes stage IV, and they recommended that these are the best groups that will benefit from arthroscopy. In the study of Atteya et al. [30], which compared operative arthroscopy to arthrocentesis, they had two groups: one group treated with arthrocentesis and the other group treated with operative arthroscopy. They found improvement in both groups but with significant improvement in the operative arthroscopy group in terms of mouth opening and pain. The reason was that in operative arthroscopy, in addition to the lysis and lavage, myotomy of the lateral pterygoid will free the disc and improve its movement, and coblation of the synovitis and retrodiscal tissue, which is rich in nerve endings) will significantly decrease the pain.

TMJ arthroscopy is an effective procedure for treating patients with internal derangement regarding pain and mouth opening.

2.8 Complications

TMJ arthroscopy is a minimally invasive procedure that is considered safe and reliable procedure. It requires a high learning curve from the surgeons to prevent the occurrence of complications, especially for levels II and III. Greene et al. [31] described the important anatomical structures to be taken in consideration during arthroscopic surgery. The facial nerve, especially the temporal branch, the neurovascular complex of the superficial temporal vessels, and the auriculotemporal nerve are close to the site of the first and second puncture. In addition to this, the glenoid fossa bone is thin, and the external auditory canal is present near the temporomandibular joint; thus, they are at risk for perforations by the trocar during puncture. This may explain why the complications of TMJ arthroscopy are usually related to the anatomy surrounding the puncture areas. It is important that every surgeon who will do this procedure should understand the complications that can occur and how to prevent and deal with them if they happen. If the surgeon is not well trained and will do this procedure, he will probably do multiple punctures trying to get inside the joint and multiple punctures trying to insert the second cannula by the triangulation technique, and this will induce more complications and iatrogenic injury. So, if you are a beginner and you tried a couple of times and you cannot place your trocar in the correct way, please abort the procedure and convert it to open surgery, as doing the open surgery in a correct way is much better than doing TMJ arthroscopy in a way that can harm the patient.

2.8.1 Extravasation of irrigation fluid outside the joint

This is usually the most common complication. Fluid usually extravasate to the temporal, parotid and masseteric regions. It usually happens as a result of copious irrigation of fluid inside the joint and also due to multiple trials of puncture, which makes multiple holes in the joint capsule through which the fluid extravasate. Usually, it resolves spontaneously in 48–72 hours. It can be prevented by controlling the amount of fluid irrigation and avoiding multiple punctures. Sometimes, extravasation of fluid could reach the medial masticatory space and the parapharyngeal space, and this could compromise the airway and require ICU admission. This usually happens by puncture of the medial wall of the joint capsule.

2.8.2 Bleeding

Bleeding is the second most frequent complication. It can occur outside the joint due to injury of the superficial temporal vessels or intraarticular, usually from the lateral pterygoid muscle during the myotomy (if the myotomy is deeper in the muscle). The problem with intraarticular bleeding is that it interferes with the vision inside the joint, making it very difficult to control the bleeding. Whenever bleeding happens, it can be controlled by compression and irrigation of cold ringer solution inside the joint till the source of bleeding is visualized, and it can be stopped using the coblator. If this cannot be done, bleeding can be stopped with a Fogarty catheter inserted inside the joint, and its balloon is inflated. Otherwise, the arthroscopy procedure is aborted, and the joint is opened surgically to stop the bleeding.

2.8.3 Damage to intraarticular structures

The damage to the intraarticular structure can be caused by disc perforation, damage to the articular eminence and fossa, and the joint capsule. This is usually caused by vigorous manipulation of instruments inside the joint, especially among inexperienced surgeons, or due to breakage of instruments inside the joint. The instruments used in TMJ arthroscopy are fine and delicate and can be broken easily with improper manipulation. This can be prevented by training the surgeons on the procedure using a special simulator or cadaver and by checking the instruments thoroughly before the procedure. In case of instrument breakage inside the joint, we should keep the instruments in view by the arthroscopy and try to extract them outside using a grasper. If this fails, we convert the procedure to open surgery and extract the piece.

2.8.4 Neurological complications

Neurological complications can be central or peripheral. The incidence in the literature ranges from 0.75 to 3.9% [2]. The central neurological complication can happen by iatrogenic injury to the glenoid fossa by the sharp trocar, causing a perforation and probably brain injury. The peripheral one usually affects the auriculotemporal nerve, the infraorbital nerve, the lingual nerve, the inferior alveolar nerve and the facial nerve or one of its branches. This complication usually happens due to repeated puncture, use of monopolar diathermy, fluid extravasation or excessive manipulation. The injury of auriculotemporal nerve usually leads to gustatory sweating, which is known as Frey's syndrome. Affection of infraorbital, lingual and inferior alveolar nerve is usually due to extravasation of fluid, especially in the parapharyngeal space. The facial nerve, especially the temporal branch, is usually affected by multiple punctures. Neurological complications are usually temporary and are getting better with time.

2.8.5 Otological complications

The ear canal, the middle ear, and the tympanic membrane are in close proximity to the TMJ which makes them liable for injury during puncture. Their incidence is usually low usually from 0.3 to 1% [2]. They are usually present in the form of blood or lacerations in the external auditory canal. Infection of the inner ear could happen if a fistula occurs between the TMJ and the inner ear. If the fistula is small, it usually closes spontaneously without problem; if it is large, it will lead to a chronic infection that requires surgical treatment.

2.8.6 Cardiological complications

This usually happens if we use epinephrine with the irrigation solution inside the joint and be absorbed into the systemic circulation. It can lead to arrhythmias, tachycardia or ventricular extrasystoles. Cardiac depression has been referred to in the literature as the result of the stimulation of the trigeminal nerve. In fact, subsequent cardiac dysfunction is caused by the stimulation of the vagus nerve via the central nucleus of the vagus nerve, which receives the afferent fibers of the fifth nerve. It is like the more frequently reported oculocardiac reflex. Although extremely rare, this complication may compromise vital parameters. A total interruption of the arthroscopic maneuvers and the rapid intervention of the anesthesiologist is mandatory to reestablish patient parameters [32].

2.8.7 Infection

It is rare with TMJ arthroscopy, and the incidence in the literature is between 0 and 1%. [2] can be prevented with prophylactic antibiotics and proper sterilization of the instruments.

2.8.8 Occlusal alterations

It consists of a posterior open bite on the ipsilateral joint secondary to postoperative edema inside the joint. It usually resolves in a few weeks. In patients with significant postoperative occlusal changes, which usually happens in level III, a splint was recommended. It was designed to raise the bite and prevent contact between upper and lower incisors and canines. Due to the resulting distalization of the bite force, joint loading was reduced, which contributed to the joint's rehabilitation. The appliance was left in place around the clock during the first 10 postoperative days and then used at night for four additional weeks.

2.8.9 Complications secondary to thermal effect

This happens sometimes with the use of laser or monopolar diathermy. The laser used inside the joint is recommended in pulse mode, as the use of continuous mode has a risk of destroying the tissue inside the joint and penetrating surrounding tissues. [2] The use of monopolar diathermy generates more heat than radiofrequency, and this could harm the chondrocyte inside the joint and can also affect the facial nerve indirectly if the current contacts the cannula. To avoid this complication, it is preferable to use radiofrequency as a source of energy such as the coblator.

After mentioning the complications, we can see that their incidence is very low and can be avoided easily with an experienced surgeon and good instrumentation. Thus, TMJ arthroscopy can be performed safely.

3. Conclusions

- TMJ arthroscopy is a safe and reliable surgical procedure for the treatment of internal derangement of the TMJ.
- It is three levels according to the procedure done, with the easiest one being level I and the hardest one being level III.
- It requires a high learning curve by the surgeons and good-quality instruments.
- Surgeons should know well the arthroscopic anatomy of the TMJ the important landmarks, and the instruments used in arthroscopy before doing the procedure.
- Beginner surgeons should perform level I perfectly and then shift to level II, and after a considerable time, when they are doing level II perfectly, they can think about level III.
- Levels II and III usually require a 30-degree lens, and level III usually requires a customized special instrument.
- The coblator is the best energy source to be used inside the joint.
- Results are excellent in the majority of patients regarding mouth opening and pain, and the best group that benefits from this procedure are patients with Wilkes stage IV.
- Complications of TMJ arthroscopy are rare and can be avoided with an experienced surgeon and good instrumentation.
- It is better to do a minimally invasive open joint surgery instead of doing an aggressive and harmful TMJ arthroscopy procedure by an inexperienced surgeon.

Acknowledgements

I want to express my deep appreciation to the Maxillofacial and Plastic Surgery department, Faculty of Dentistry, Alexandria University, Egypt, for facilitating the work of TMJ arthroscopy in the department and for the extreme eagerness to buy all the instruments needed for this procedure. I express my deepest gratitude to Prof. Dr. Florencio Monje Gil, Professor of Oral and Maxillofacial Surgery, University Hospital of Badajoz, Badajoz, Spain, for his great support, guidance, and advice in learning TMJ arthroscopy. He taught me a lot about the management of these cases and the skills of operative procedures. I want to thank also doctor Raúl Gonzalez Garcia, consultant of Oral and Maxillofacial Surgery, University Hospital la princesa, Madrid, Spain, for his help and support and for giving me the chance to learn from his experience in the TMJ arthroscopy.

Conflict of interest

I have no conflict of interest to declare.

Author details

Aly Mohamed Atteya
Maxillofacial and Plastic Surgery, Faculty of Dentistry, Alexandria University, Egypt

*Address all correspondence to: aly.atteya@alexu.edu.eg

References

[1] McCain JP. Principles and practice of temporomandibular joint arthroscopy. Operative Dentistry. 1996;**333**:169-194

[2] Monje, Gil F. Surgical Management of Temporomandibular Joint: Vol. 1 Arthroscopy. Apple Books, I tunes; 2014

[3] Onishi M. Arthroscopy of the temporomandibular joint (author's transl). Kokubyo Gakkai Zasshi. The Journal of the Stomatological Society, Japan. 1975;**42**(2):207-213

[4] Hilsabeck RB, Laskin DM. Arthroscopy of the temporomandibular joint of the rabbit. Journal of Oral Surgery (American Dental Association: 1965). 1978;**36**(12):938-943

[5] Murakami K, Hoshino K. Regional anatomical nomenclature and arthroscopic terminology in human temporomandibular joints. Okajimas Folia Anatomica Japonica. 1982;**58**:745-760

[6] McCain JP. Arthroscopy of the human temporomandibular joint. Journal of Oral and Maxillofacial Surgery. 1988;**46**:648-655

[7] Sanders B. Arthroscopic surgery of the temporomandibular joint: Treatment of internal derangement with persistent closed lock. Oral Surgery, Oral Medicine, and Oral Pathology. 1986;**62**:361-372

[8] Murakami K, Ono T. Temporomandibular joint arthroscopy by inferolateral approach. International Journal of Oral and Maxillofacial Surgery. 1986;**15**:410-417

[9] McCain JP, Podrasky AE, Zabiegalski NA. Arthroscopic disc repositioning and suturing: A preliminary report. Journal of Oral and Maxillofacial Surgery. 1992;**50**(6):568-579

[10] Yang C, Cai XY, Chen MJ, Zhang SY. New arthroscopic disc repositioning and suturing technique for treating an anteriorly displaced disc of the temporomandibular joint: Part I--technique introduction. International Journal of Oral and Maxillofacial Surgery. 2012;**41**:1058-1063

[11] Martín-Granizo R, Millón-Cruz A. Discopexy using resorbable pins in temporomandibular joint arthroscopy: Clinical and magnetic resonance imaging medium-term results. Journal of Cranio-Maxillofacial Surgery. 2016;**44**(4):479-486

[12] González-García R, Usandizaga JL, Rodríguez-Campo FJ. Arthroscopic anatomy and lysis and lavage of the temporomandibular joint. Atlas of the Oral and Maxillofacial Surgery Clinics of North America. 2011;**19**(2):131-144

[13] Holmlund A, Gynther G, Axelsson S. Efficacy of arthroscopic lysis and lavage in patients with chronic locking of the temporomandibular joint. International Journal of Oral and Maxillofacial Surgery. 1994;**23**(5):262-265

[14] Sanders B. Management of internal derangements of the temporomandibular joint. Seminars in Orthodontics. 1995;**1**(4):244-257

[15] Al-Moraissi EA, Wolford LM, Ellis E 3rd, Neff A. The hierarchy of different treatments for arthrogenous temporomandibular disorders: A network meta-analysis of randomized clinical trials. Journal of Cranio-Maxillo-Facial Surgery. 2020;**48**:9-23

[16] Nitzan DW, Dolwick MF, Heft MW. Arthroscopic lavage and lysis of the temporomandibular joint: A change in perspective. Journal of Oral and Maxillofacial Surgery. 1990;**48**(8):798-801

[17] Indresano T. Arthroscopic surgery of the temporomandibular joint. Journal of Oral and Maxillofacial Surgery. 1989;**47**:439

[18] Montgomery M, Van Sickels J, Harm S. Arthroscopic TMJ surgery: Effects on signs, symptoms and disc position. Journal of Oral and Maxillofacial Surgery. 1989;**47**:1263

[19] Moses JJ, Sartoris D, Glass R, Tanaka T, Poker I. The effect of arthroscopic surgical lysis and lavage of the superior joint space on TMJ disc position and mobility. Journal of Oral and Maxillofacial Surgery. 1989;**47**(7):674-678

[20] Moses JJ, Poker ID. TMJ arthroscopic surgery: An analysis of 237 patients. Journal of Oral and Maxillofacial Surgery: Official Journal of the American Association of Oral and Maxillofacial Surgeons. 1989;**47**(8):790-794

[21] Israel HA, Roser SM. Patient response to temporomandibular joint arthroscopy: Preliminary findings in 24 patients. Journal of Oral and Maxillofacial Surgery. 1989;**47**(6):570-573

[22] Clark GT, Moody DG, Sanders B. Arthroscopic treatment of temporomandibular joint locking resulting from disc derangement: Two-year results. Journal of Oral and Maxillofacial Surgery. 1991;**49**(2):157-164

[23] Clark GT, Sanders B, Bertolami CN. Advances in diagnostic and surgical arthroscopy of the temporomandibular joint. Implant Dentistry. 1993;**2**(2):136

[24] Machoň V, Šedý J, Klíma K, Hirjak D, Foltán R. Arthroscopic lysis and lavage in patients with temporomandibular anterior disc displacement without reduction. International Journal of Oral and Maxillofacial Surgery. 2012;**41**(1):109-113

[25] Ahmed N, Sidebottom A, O'Connor M, Kerr HL. Prospective outcome assessment of the therapeutic benefits of arthroscopy and arthrocentesis of the temporomandibular joint. British Journal of Oral and Maxillofacial Surgery. 2012;**50**(8):745-748

[26] Murakami KI, Tsuboi Y, Bessho K, Yokoe Y, Nishida M, Iizuka T. Outcome of arthroscopic surgery to the temporomandibular joint correlates with stage of internal derangement: Five-year follow-up study. British Journal of Oral and Maxillofacial Surgery. 1998;**36**(1):30-34

[27] Moses JJ, Topper DC. A functional approach to the treatment of temporomandibular joint internal derangement. Journal of Craniomandibular Disorders. 1991;**5**(1):19-27

[28] Zhang SY, Liu XM, Yang C, Cai XY, Chen MJ, Haddad MS, et al. New arthroscopic disc repositioning and suturing technique for treating internal derangement of the temporomandibular joint: Part II—Magnetic resonance imaging evaluation. Journal of Oral and Maxillofacial Surgery. 2010;**68**(8):1813-1817

[29] González-García R, Rodríguez-Campo FJ. Arthroscopic lysis and lavage versus operative arthroscopy in the outcome of temporomandibular

joint internal derangement: A comparative study based on Wilkes stages. Journal of Oral and Maxillofacial Surgery. 2011;**69**(10):2513-2524

[30] Atteya AM, Warda MH, Fata MM, Medra AM, Gil FM. Prospective randomized study between arthrocentesis and operative arthroscopy in the management of temporomandibular joint internal derangement. Alexandria Dental Journal. 2021;**46**(1):58-65

[31] Greene MW, Hackney FL, Van Sickels JE. Arthroscopy of the temporomandibular joint: An anatomic perspective. Journal of Oral and Maxillofacial Surgery. 1989;**47**(4):386-389

[32] González-García R, Rodríguez-Campo FJ, Escorial-Hernández V, Muñoz-Guerra MF, Sastre-Pérez J, Naval-Gías L, et al. Complications of temporomandibular joint arthroscopy: A retrospective analytic study of 670 arthroscopic procedures. Journal of Oral and Maxillofacial Surgery. 2006;**64**(11):1587-1591

Chapter 5

ICR: Idiopathic Condylar Resorption

Michal Beňo

Abstract

Idiopathic condylar resorption (ICR) is a localized, non-inflammatory degenerative disease of the temporomandibular joint (TMJ) characterized by osteolysis that leads to the destruction of the mandibular condyles. The etiology of ICR is still unknown. Possible risk factors have already been identified, including orthognathic surgery. This condition is more common in women than men. Radiographic study in these cases indicates a diminished condylar head volume, decreased ramus height, change in condylar shape, and progressive Class II basal bone relationship. Computed tomography (CT) and cone beam computed tomography (CBCT) are suitable for diagnosing initial ICR manifestation and progression. Drugs and occlusal splint therapy represent a conservative form of treatment. Arthroscopy and arthrocentesis can help reduce pain and improve joint function. In advanced stages of ICR, total joint replacement may be necessary. The approach to treating ICR cases should be individualized and based on the extent of the disease process. There are a number of patients with ICR who are best treated with total joint replacement (TJR).

Keywords: idiopathic condylar resorption, progressive condylar resorption, temporomandibular disorder, temporomandibular joint (TMJ) replacement, anterior open bite, orthognathic surgery, Class II

1. Introduction

Idiopathic condylar resorption (ICR) is a very rare clinical condition of unknown etiology that leads to the destruction of the mandibular condyles [1, 2]. Idiopathic condylar resorption (ICR) is a localized, non-inflammatory degenerative disease of the temporomandibular joint (TMJ) characterized by osteolysis of the mandibular condyl [3]. ICR should be treated and considered as a diagnosis excluding other resorptions [1].

Idiopathic condylar resorption is a well-known but poorly understood disease process with an incidence ratio in women and men of 9:1. ICR incidence is approximately one in 5000 patients or about one to two per orthodontic office [4, 5].

Since it overwhelmingly affects adolescent girls and young women in their second and third decades of life, Wolford et al. termed it "cheerleader syndrome" [2, 6–9].

This degenerative disease is alternately known as condylysis, condylar atrophy, condylar hypoplasia, progressive condylar resorption (PCR), aggressive condylar resorption, and postorthognathic condylar resorption [6, 8–12].

The condition can lead to progressive and irreversible reduction in mandible volume and height, usually bilaterally, which can worsen a retrognathic face. If only one joint is affected, there is a deviation of the chin and the lower dental midline to the affected side and facial asymmetry. More often, however, we observe bilateral changes. There is shortening of the vertical height of the ramus of the mandible, counterclockwise (CCW) rotation, progression of the skeletal Class II, and anterior open bite.

It can also lead to a reduction in the translucency of the oropharyngeal airways in severe cases. In growing patients, ICR primarily manifests as impaired growth of the lower jaw, along with anterior disc dislocation [5, 8–11].

2. Etiology

In most cases, there is no clearly identifiable cause, and therefore, the condition is generally referred to as ICR. Patients were only identified as having adolescent ICR if no autoimmune disease was present and there was no previous facial trauma, TMJ compression, or other pathological conditions affecting the TMJ. They underwent standard diagnostic examination by a pediatric rheumatologist [6, 13].

Risk factors that play significant roles in ICR etiology include:

excessive functional loading of the TMJ—ICR could arise after increased mechanical loading on the temporomandibular joints (TMJ) caused by: (1) occlusal changes (orthognathic surgery, orthodontics, prosthodontic dentures); (2) an internal TMJ derangement; (3) TMJ parafunction; (4) trauma (e.g., condylar fracture); and/or (5) unstable occlusion [4, 6, 9, 14].

Arnett et al. described that ICR occurs as a result of dysfunctional remodeling, which may occur as a result of (a) reduced adaptive capacity of joint structures or (b) extreme mechanical loading of the TMJs that exceeds their adaptive capacity [7, 15, 16].

Orthognathic surgical risk factors include the use of maxillomandibular fixation after surgery, a large gonial angle of the mandibular plane, being an adolescent or young female (aged 11–30), a retrognathic mandible, a short ramus, a posteriorly inclined condylar neck, and reduced condyle height or volume. All of these are likely to cause adverse joint loading [2, 10, 16].

A healthy TMJ undergoing natural remodeling can withstand and adapt to high mechanical loads, including parafunctional habits, such as nighttime bruxism, orthodontic treatment, and the wearing of elastics and orthotic appliances, such as a Herbst appliance or chin strap. Facial trauma and orthognathic surgical procedures can also cause increased TMJ loading [5, 15, 16].

The development of condylar resorption in young adult women can occur with excessive mechanical stress on the TMJ structures when the adaptive capacity is exceeded. Studies indicate severe trauma or bilateral sagittal split osteotomy (BSSO) advancement more than 15 mm as the cause. For example, Scheerlink et al. showed that significant surgical displacement of the mandible led to patients developing significant condylar resorption. In these cases, it appears the forces produced by the stretched muscles and soft tissues exceed the adaptive capacity of the joints [5, 15–17].

The hormonal influence of estrogen and prolactin and their influence on bone turnover are investigated based on the presence of estrogen receptors in the human TMJ.

Due to estrogen receptors and the bilateral occurrence of degenerative processes, the subject of investigation is a low level of estrogens affecting the metabolism of TMJ cartilage and bone, as well as a possible genetic predisposition [6, 10, 18–20].

Gunson et al. demonstrated low serum 17 beta-estradiol levels to be a major factor in progressive condylar resorption. They report that the use of oral contraceptives and abnormal menstrual cycles are often seen in women with severe condylar resorption. Milam reports that low estrogen levels can have a negative effect on joint tissues [5, 21, 22].

Several clinical studies have shown that serum 17 beta-estradiol levels, either at midcycle or at the follicular phase, are abnormally low in patients with ICR. Although the specific causes of ICR are unclear, hormonal imbalance is likely one of several factors responsible for its etiopathogenesis [23].

Yuan et al. in this study did not observe any uniqueness regarding irregular menstrual cycles, use of oral contraceptives, or use of other menstrual-related medications in patients with ICR.

Given that irregular menstrual cycles occur in women in the general population as well as in adolescent girls not long after menarche, venous blood was drawn and analyzed between days 2 and 5 of menstruation to minimize variability. However, the study results did not demonstrate aberrant serum 17 beta-estradiol levels in either women or men, or in patients with ICR [23].

The patients in the study had a standard age of onset of puberty and menarche, the use of oral contraceptives was not the cause of ICR progression, and there were no differences between the patients in estradiol levels and regularity of the menstrual cycle [23].

Other risk factors include nutritional deficiencies (e.g., vitamin D and omega-3 fatty acids), preexisting degenerative joint disease, genetic predisposition (matrix metalloproteinase (MMP) polymorphisms, vitamin D receptors, aromatase, and estrogen receptors), reduced ability of the joint area to remodel, for example, due to advanced age, systemic diseases (autoimmune, endocrine, and metabolic), and/or the inhibitory effect of low concentrations of certain sex hormones (especially estrogens) [1].

Risk factors can generally be divided into two categories: patient-related and surgery-related.

Patient-related risk factors include age, gender, medications, systemic disorders, mandibular anatomy, bone density, and dental occlusion. The population includes young women with skeletal malocclusion II class, with mandibular retrognathism and an anterior open bite, and a slender backward-inclined condylar neck [6].

Risks related to surgery include: Medial or lateral condylar torque with rigid fixation of the mandibular segments during surgery, prolonged maxillomandibular fixation, counterclockwise rotation in orthognathic surgery, and large displacements of the mandible. The detailed ICR onset and progression mechanism remains controversial, and the current treatment principles are based on empirical belief and tradition rather than science. It is difficult for a single observer to assemble a large enough group of ICR patients to support a statistically significant treatment study. It is challenging to prevent ICR and give an accurate prognosis [2, 9, 13, 14, 20, 23].

From the point of view of progression, we distinguish between active and stable forms of ICR. The manifestations of ICR are clinically similar to those of other diseases of joint structures such as osteoarthritis and juvenile idiopathic arthritis (JIA) of the TMJ. As the two conditions progress in quite different ways, and require different therapeutic approaches, early differential diagnosis is crucial [1, 2, 13].

Two categories of TMJ remodeling can occur: functional and dysfunctional remodeling. Functional TMJ remodeling involves morphological changes in joint structures not associated with any significant joint changes or occlusion.

Therefore, functional remodeling is characterized by stable mandibular ramus height, stable occlusion, and normal growth. Dysfunctional remodeling is characterized by morphological change of the TMJ (reduced condylar head volume), reduced mandibular branch height, progressive mandibular retrusion, or reduced growth. The effects of dysfunctional remodeling (condylar resorption) on the growing mandible are obvious: When it occurs during growth, it reduces condyle size and mandible growth rate, leading to mandibular retrusion, with a lack of full anterior growth [11].

3. Diagnostics

With the development of radiological technology, ICR is now classified primarily based on changes in condyle morphology. There is strong demand for a more practical classification of ICR. In this study, ICRs with different degrees of bone loss were investigated using a three-dimensional (3D) reconstruction technique. Individual subgroups of ICR include: ICR I moderate resorption; ICR II resorption that exceeded the maximum transverse diameter of the condyle; and ICR III, when the condylar head showed a change in normal morphology [14].

The articular process has a layer of connective cartilage on its surface. When the cartilage breaks down, the outer bony surface of the head is absorbed [24, 25]. On imaging examination, this manifests itself as resorption lacunae with the disappearance of the bony cortical layer. Other changes include a change in the volume of the condylar process and a reduction and shortening of the mandibular ramus. Resorption changes can occur not only in the area of the condyle but also in the articular eminence, which tends to flatten. These degenerative bone changes are often accompanied by pain (**Figure 1**) [5, 26, 27].

In the diagnosis of ICR, resorption is rapid, and progression generally long-term. ICR progression can cause occlusion and musculature to become unstable, leading to maxillofacial deformity, dysfunction, and TMJ pain [9, 18, 20].

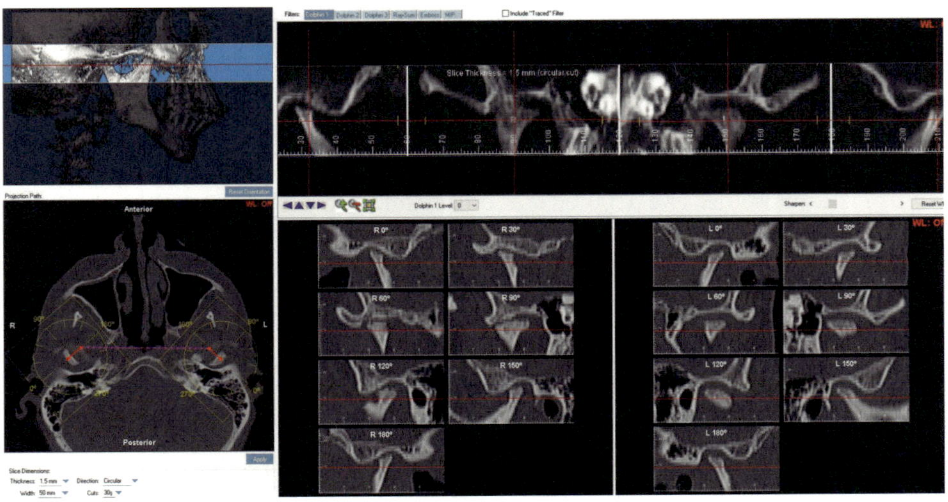

Figure 1.
CT scans and detailed view of the joint.

4. Gender and age

Interestingly, there is sometimes an unexplained "burnout" of the resorption process when a woman is in her mid-20s, although resorption can extend into the early 30s. We do not recommend orthognathic surgery for adolescent girls with suspected ICR [5].

Current findings suggest that estrogen prompted increased bone resorption on the anterior surface of the condylar head in rabbit models at an early stage, whereas TMJ function restoration occurred in a normal manner [28].

An animal study by Wu et al. found that mechanical stress (resin buildup on the right molars) applied to the mandible in estrogen-deficient mice led to more extensive condylar degeneration compared to mice with normal estrogen levels. Mice with low serum 17 betaestradiol levels had the lowest cartilage thickness and the highest degree of osteoarthritis (osteoclastic activity and apoptosis) during histological analysis. In cell culture, the authors showed that estradiol increases micro-RNA (miRNA) expression and suppresses hyaluronan levels, which are thought to protect the joint. These findings further suggest a role for serum 17 beta-estradiol levels as a factor in ICR development. However, there is no test or biomarker to determine which cases will progress and which will remain quiescent [8].

5. Assessment of the maxillofacial skeleton

When assessing skeletal structures, no significant differences were found between the ICR and control groups in terms of the position of the maxilla relative to the skull base [20].

Vertical assessment of the maxillofacial skeleton indicated that N= nasion, A= A-point maxila, upper facial height, was not significantly different in the ICR group compared to the control group. Meanwhile, lower facial height was significantly greater in the ICR group compared to the control group. Mandible size in the ICR group was significantly smaller than in the control group, in terms of both mandibular body length and branch height. Excessive gonial angle and significant clockwise rotation of the mandible were observed in patients with ICR, causing a downward movement of the B point. Mandibular condylar resorption in ICR causes a reduction in the volume and height of the mandibular condyle, leading to mandibular retrusion [20].

One third of patients with ICR had orthodontic treatment before the diagnosis of ICR. These findings suggest that although the mechanical force used in orthodontic treatment on the TMJ is negligible under normal conditions, it may be associated with the development and progression of ICR [4].

Internal TMJ derangement with disc dislocation is considered an intrinsic factor, whereas surgical displacement of the mandible contributes to ICR onset as an extrinsic factor. Mandibular orthognathic surgical advancement (BSSO) may contribute to the development of ICR, but it is not sufficient to induce ICR [4]. The size and shape of the condyles were significantly different in patients with ICR on CT (**Figures 2** and **3**) [5]. In a study by Iwasa et al., they observed the distribution of stress in the TMJ during muscle contraction on 3D models and concluded that more stress is concentrated on the lateral and anterior parts of the condyle surface. Similarly, more pressure is exerted laterally than medially and anteriorly than posteriorly on the condyle during mouth opening. Remodeling in these areas differs from each other [4]. CT examination must

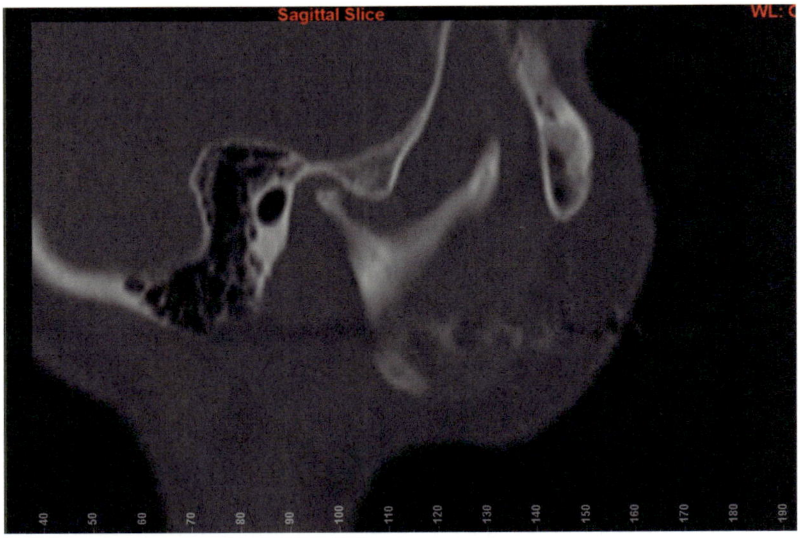

Figure 2.
CT scan in sagittal view.

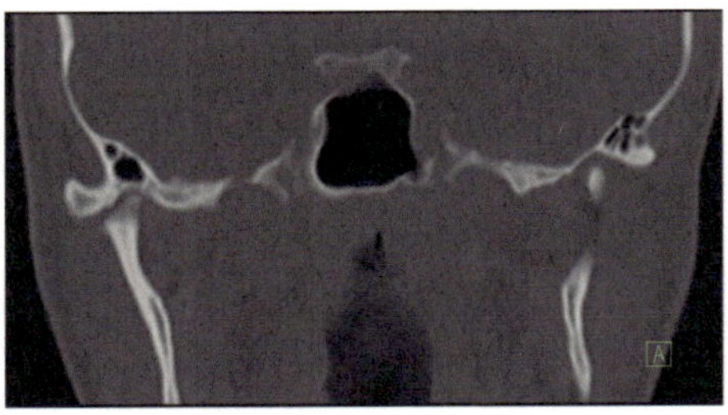

Figure 3.
CT scan in coronal view.

be performed in growing patients with suspected ICR, because condyle shape changes and condyle size reduction may precede clinical findings. This can contribute to the detection of ICR and early treatment initiation. Magnetic resonance imaging (MRI) findings may provide detailed information on disc location and soft structure [4].

6. Orthognathic surgery as a risk factor

Orthognathic surgery to correct open bite malocclusion includes Le Fort I osteotomy surgery on the maxilla and BSSO of the mandible along with CCW rotation of the entire maxillomandibular complex (**Figure 4**). Surgical advancement of the jaws causes a sudden change in the position of the condyles in the fossa and thus the loading of the TMJ. Functional remodeling will occur in most patients, but in some the condyles are overloaded and begin to resorb [5, 15].

Arnett et al. demonstrated that the use of bicortical screws to fix segments during BSSO can rotate the condylar segments either laterally or medially in the glenoid fossa. This inappropriate seating and condyle fixation could initiate condylar resorption. To minimize this, they recommend using titanium bone plates adapted to the

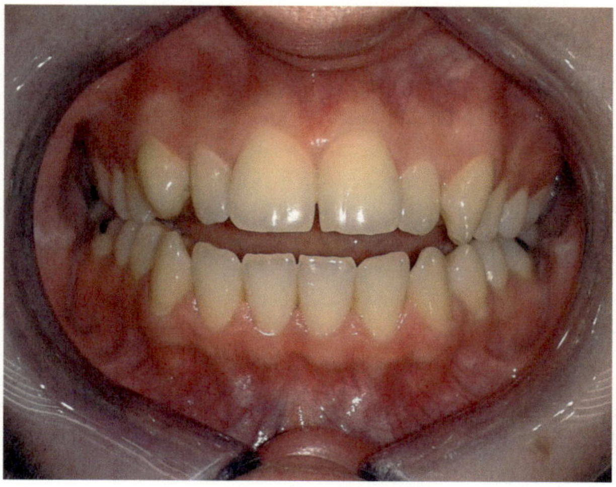

Figure 4.
Anterior open bite (AOB).

outer cortical surfaces of both segments with monocortical screw fixation. They also point out that overseating the condyle in the fossa during BSSO can cause compression, resulting in dysfunctional joint remodeling [15, 16].

Most orthognathic surgical procedures can result in gross mandibular condyle positional changes, so these procedures come with a high risk of gross condylar morphologic changes. They found that intraoperative condylar torquing or posteriorization leads to condylar resorption and late mandibular relapse [11].

Parafunction can cause joint compression, in turn increasing joint resorption. It can increase intracapsular pressure and inhibit capillary perfusion, causing ischemic damage with accompanying loss of temporomandibular tissue volume leading to mandibular retrusion. By definition, unstable occlusion occurs when the teeth intercuspidate by muscular force, and the condyle is displaced and/or compressed. The compressed position of the joint will then cause some degree of remodeling to occur, depending on the magnitude of the position change and coexisting systemic factors [11].

Drugs and occlusal splint therapy represent a conservative form of treatment. The therapeutic effects of the splint should minimize the risk of pressure-related resorption progression [25]. We achieve this by proper condylar seating, adaptation of the osteosynthetic plate, and the use of monocortical screws, the use of a postoperative splint. Postoperative treatment includes medication, mouth opening rehabilitation, and class II elastic bands [7, 11, 16, 29, 30].

Specific cytokines and enzymes are involved in the degradation of the bone mass of the mandibular condyle. By blocking cytokines and enzymes, we can prevent the progression of condylar resorption. Tumor necrosis factor-alpha (TNF-α) promotes osteoclastogenesis and the activity of osteoclasts in the patient's joints. By administering TNF-α inhibitors, we can minimize bone loss in the mandibular condyle. Another enzyme is the matrix metalloproteinase (MMP) that breaks down collagen. Tetracyclines as MMP inhibitors reduce joint erosion in susceptible patients.

Patients with preexisting signs of ICR before orthognathic surgery had unfavorable outcomes. Arnett and Tumborello reported that four out of nine of these patients had postoperative condylar resorption [13], while Huang et al. reported that four out of 18 had postoperative relapse [5].

In a study by Hoppenreijs et al., condylar resorption incidence in patients with ICR after maxillary surgery to correct Class II open bite malocclusions was lower than after surgery involving both jaws (9% versus 23%) [25].

ICR treatment depends on the activity of the disease and condyle resorption severity. When there is inactivity, and sufficient condylar mass is preserved providing a reliable centric relationship with respect to the jaws, routine orthognathic surgery can be considered. If the disease is active, then condyle reconstruction with autogenous or alloplastic material is necessary [2].

7. Differential diagnosis

Alimanovic et al. in his study showed a high degree of overlap between the radiological and clinical manifestations of TMJ in patients with JIA and ICR. The diagnostic distinction between these two conditions remains challenging, especially in JIA patients with isolated TMJ involvement and no involvement of other joints [31].

The active phase resorption usually occurs after the completion of jaw growth, which is not affected. Painless but adequate temporomandibular joint function and mandibular range of motion are assumed [32].

JIA occurs between the ages of seven and 14, and TMJ involvement is more likely to negatively affect mandibular growth than ICR, leading to secondary deformity of the jaw [33].

7.1 The role of the TMJ disc

The TMJ disc acts as a shock absorber during mandibular movements, while allowing smooth translational and rotational movements [5].

Wolford and Cardenas recommend joint replacement surgery to attach the dislocated disc to the condyle head before or during orthognathic surgery for ICR to prevent disc dislocation recurrence or disc morphology changes. Other surgeons disagree and claim that disc surgery is necessary. When performing orthognathic surgery in patients with ICR, they do not enter the joint, especially if the joint is functional and the condition progression-free, even if the condyle and ramus are affected by the disease [5, 16, 24, 33].

We should note that TMJ disc dislocation occurs in about one third of asymptomatic individuals in the population, whereas ICR is relatively rare [5].

7.2 Incidence

Group of orthodontists confirmed the rarity of occurrence by reporting an average of 1.3 ICR cases in their careers. Surgical centers that perform a large number of orthognathic procedures report an incidence of 2–5%, which is still rare [5].

Early symptoms and signs of condylar resorption are subtle. Resorption is usually slow, at approximately 1.0–1.5 mm per year, so it may initially be difficult to clinically identify [6, 9, 13].

7.3 Diagnosing patients with ICR

The patient should be evaluated for estrogen and rheumatoid factor levels.

According to the literature, resorption after orthognathic surgery is evident in two-dimensional imaging no earlier than 6 months and no later than 2 years after surgery. According to the international literature, both computed tomography (CT) and cone beam computed tomography (CBCT) are suitable for diagnosing initial ICR manifestation and progression. The consensus is that three-dimensional imaging (CT/CBCT) is the current diagnostic standard for imaging and documenting the extent of ICR [1, 3].

Another imaging technique is scintigraphy. The potential benefit of scintigraphy in distinguishing between active and steady-state resorption has been critically evaluated by some authors [1].

7.4 Orthopantomograms and lateral cephalometric radiographs

An orthopantomogram (OPG) can be used for basic examination of the condylar anatomy. In ICR patients, an OPG will show whether the condyle has lost bone mass relative to the rest of the mandible, as it will appear thin or shortened with a flattened capitulum. The condylar neck will often have a distal slope (**Figure 5**) [5].

7.5 Magnetic resonance imaging (MRI)

Magnetic resonance imaging (MRI) is useful for examining TMJ soft tissues and determining the cartilaginous integrity of the condylar surfaces, the position and condition of the articular disc, joint effusion, and bone marrow edema. However, it does not provide diagnostic images of the condylar cortex or eminence, which are clearly defined by CBCT scanning [5].

7.6 Occlusal splints: diagnostic aspects

Occlusal orthodontic splints are suggested as a joint stabilization modality in cases of ICR for joint pain and dysfunction, and also prior to orthognathic surgery.

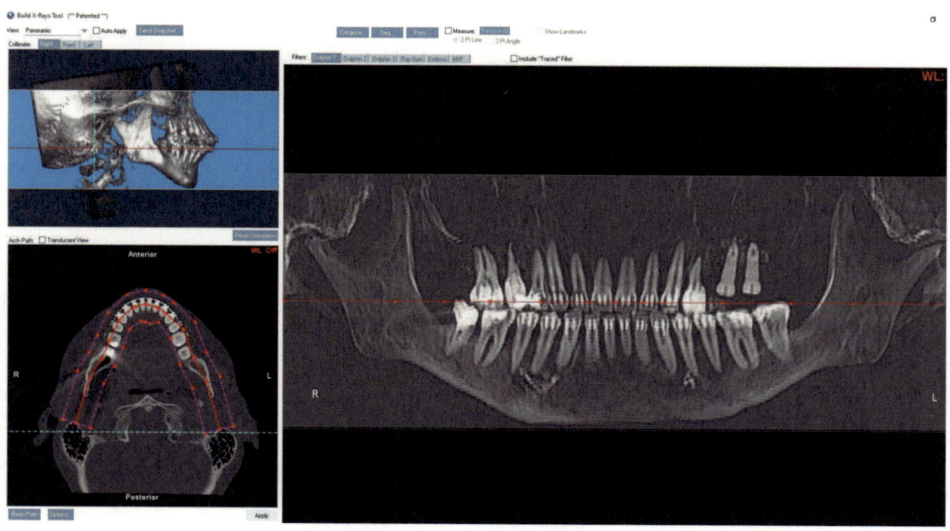

Figure 5.
OPG distal inclination of the condyle.

A maxillary occlusal splint should be routinely placed at the time of retention for TMJ comfort after orthognathic/orthodontic treatment in order to reduce forces on the joint, and to evaluate the stability of the correction [5, 21, 33].

8. Treatment

If we know the underlying disease that is evidently the cause of condylar resorption, we must treat it adequately. If we do not know the cause, even with ICR, we can start with conservative treatment. We manage the symptoms and treatment can slow the progression of the disease [1].

Zhou et al. in a study have shown that stabilizing splint therapy can reduce mechanical overloading of the TMJ, slow bone destruction, and promote condylar remodeling. Conservative therapeutic measures include functional therapy (e.g., occlusal splints), adjunctive orthodontic treatment, physiotherapy, and pharmacotherapy [5].

In the case of symptomatic active condylar resorption (pain, functional problems), conservative therapeutic procedures should initially be used to suppress symptoms. In particular, traditional orthodontic options (such as removable and fixed appliances and tooth extractions) can be applied in preparation for surgical therapy. The most common surgical modalities for the treatment of ICR are: arthrocentesis, arthroplasty, condylectomy, total joint replacement TMJ-endoprosthesis [1].

An interesting muscle that inevitably has to change its insertion during the destruction of the condyle is the lateral pterygoid muscle, and its functionality changes as well. Unfortunately, we found that there is almost no literature specific to ICR that deals with the lateral pterygoid muscle, and none of it is related to MRI. Each individual case of ICR requires a specially tailored approach to surgical treatment [1].

8.1 Medications

Aspirin or non-steroidal anti-inflammatory drugs (NSAIDs) are commonly used. Muscular symptoms can be treated with muscle relaxants and rehabilitation [3].

In the field of pharmacotherapy, there are new therapeutic approaches that need to be evaluated with long-term and more extensive case studies [1].

Occlusal splint therapy may be the best strategy to stabilize the TMJ make an accurate diagnosis [3].

The most common approach is for a severe open bite to be treated through orthognathic surgery, but in some cases, temporary anchorage devices (TADs) may be indicated to facilitate orthodontic correction. Many studies have reported successful molar intrusion using orthodontic TADs to improve occlusion and facial esthetics in patients with severe anterior open bite. In our case, the patient's retrognathic profile was significantly improved by counterclockwise rotation of the mandible using multiple buccal and palatal TADs along with a double transpalatal arch. Long-term stability after anterior open bite TAD treatment has not been fully explored; however, our patient had an acceptable overbite that remained stable over a 2-year retention period [3].

Rheumatoid factor serology should be supplemented, although rheumatoid factor serologies are usually negative in patients with ICR. A history of TMJ problems and disc dislocation is an important factor—if pain is reported, it may be an indication that the disease is active [5].

Gunson and Arnett have taken a more biomedical and pharmacological approach to the treatment of patients with ICR. They prescribe an occlusal splint for 6 months before and after orthognathic surgery to reduce the mechanical load on the joint. They reported stable results after orthognathic surgery at 24-month follow-up in 24 patients with ICR [19].

The approach to treating ICR cases should be individualized and based on the extent of the disease process. There are a number of patients with ICR who are best treated with total joint replacement (TJR). These are individuals with impaired function, manifested by severely limited joint mobility; failure of previous orthognathic surgery; and poor prognosis for orthognathic surgical correction.

In individual cases, allogeneic condylar process reconstruction is combined with orthognathic surgery. It is recommended that orthognathic surgery be performed as part of a more complex reconstructive procedure along with temporomandibular joint replacement in a single-stage procedure. It should be noted that isolated orthognathic surgery (without endoprosthesis) is associated with an increased risk of recurrence, especially between 6 and 12 months after active resorption. The goal of any surgical therapy for condylar resorption is to minimize further compressive loading of the condyle [1].

9. Conclusions

In conclusion, it may be said that the goals of reconstruction in a patient with mandibular deformity and altered condylar integrity may include the following: (1) restoration of improved joint function; (2) restoration of optimal facial esthetics; (3) improvement in occlusion and long-term dental health; (4) pain relief; and often (5) simultaneous improvement in the patient's associated speech articulation, masticatory ability, and breathing difficulties [32].

Alsabban et al. reported that the management of ICR is controversial and that there are currently no published randomized clinical trials comparing the outcomes of different nonsurgical and surgical treatment options for ICR [9, 34].

Patients who underwent total joint reconstruction had 95–100% postoperative stability with follow-up times ranging from 3 months to 11 years (**Figures 6–8**) [35].

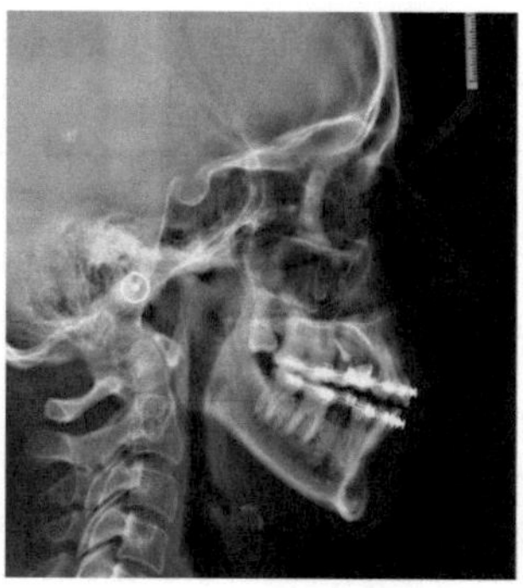

Figure 6.
X-ray patient with anterior open bite.

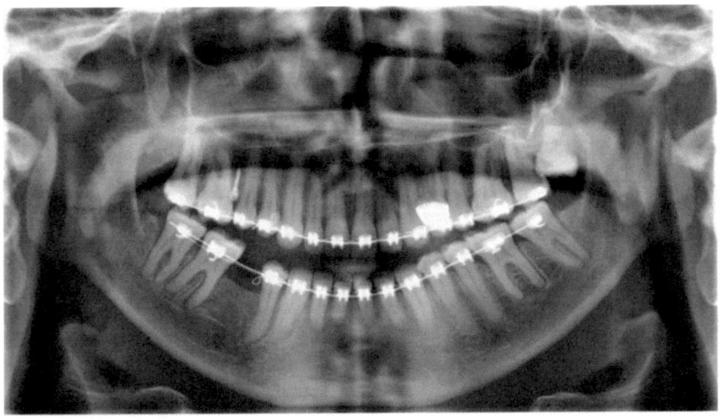

Figure 7.
OPG patient with anterior open bite.

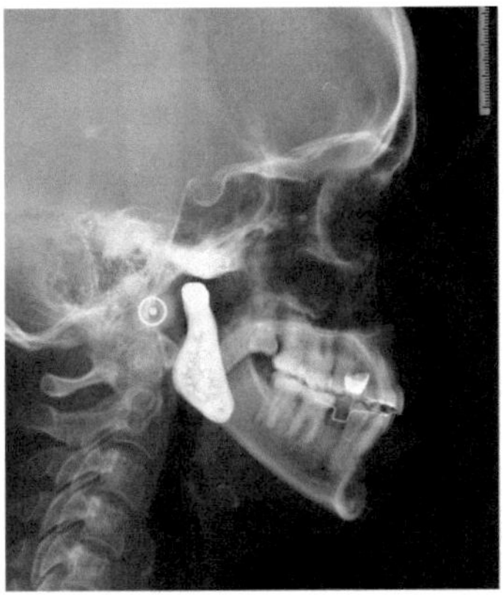

Figure 8.
X-ray patient with TMJ TJR bilateral.

9.1 Rationale for the use of TMJ TJR

Total alloplastic joint replacement is a treatment option for end-stage TMJ disease, when the joint is so architecturally devastated by disease or injury that it results in severe functional disability of the patient. The bone architecture of the joint has pathological changes that show up in imaging. In the end stage, the modern practice of orthopedic surgery would be unthinkable without TMJ TEP [5].

Reasons for using alloplastic prosthesis as the first choice in the surgical treatment of patients with ICR include: (1) elimination of the bone graft donor site, reducing morbidity and operation time; (2) no need for postoperative remodeling, so the mandibular position remains reliably stable over the long term; (3) prostheses longevity is no longer in question, as there are reports of more than 20 years of follow-up of TMJ fossae and mandibular components; and (4) these prostheses do not have the problem of unpredictable or excessive growth. There are highly predictable outcomes in relation to stability, TMJ and occlusal function, esthetics, and pain reduction [6, 7, 29, 30, 33].

The goals of jaw replacement are to: (1) improve the function and form of the mandible; (2) reduce suffering and disability; (3) contain overtreatment and costs; and (4) prevent morbidity.

The advantages of TMJ TJR are: (1) physical therapy can begin immediately; (2) there is no need for a secondary donor site, while operative time is reduced; and (3) they are able to mimic normal anatomy. For patients with ICR/PCR, an additional advantage is that the materials from which these devices are constructed are not susceptible to the pathophysiology of the disease process [5].

The etiology of ICR is still unknown. Possible risk factors have already been identified, including orthognathic surgery. Whether condylar resorptions are a consequence of orthognathic surgery, or occur in their context by mere coincidence, requires further research [1].

Acknowledgements

Author thanks to Medika Trade Praha for support.

Author details

Michal Beňo
Department of Oral Maxillofacial Surgery, Charles University and Faculty Hospital Prague, Czech Republic

*Address all correspondence to: michbeno@gmail.com

References

[1] Riechmann M, Schmidt C, Ahlers MO, Feurer I, Kleinheinz J, Kolk A, et al. Controversial aspects of diagnostics and therapy of idiopathic condylar resorption: An analysis of evidence- and consensus-based recommendations based on an interdisciplinary guideline project. Journal of Clinical Medicine. 2023;**12**:4946. DOI: 10.3390/jcm12154946

[2] Ji YD, Resnick CM, Peacock ZS. Idiopathic condylar resorption: A systematic review of etiology and management. Oral Surgery, Oral Medicine, Oral Pathology, Oral Radiology. 2020;**130**(6):632-639. DOI: 10.1016/j.oooo.2020.07.008 Epub 2020 Jul 21

[3] Lee GH, Park JH, Lee SM, Moon DN. Orthodontic treatment protocols for patients with idiopathic condylar resorption. The Journal of Clinical Pediatric Dentistry. 2019;**43**(4):292-303. DOI: 10.17796/1053-4625-43.4.12 Epub 2019 May 16

[4] Iwasa A, Tanaka E. Signs, symptoms, and morphological features of idiopathic condylar resorption in orthodontic patients: A survey-based study. Journal of Clinical Medicine. 2022;**11**(6):1552. DOI: 10.3390/jcm11061552

[5] Handelman CS, Mercuri L. Idiopathic/progressive condylar resorption: An orthodontic perspective. In: Kandasamy S, Greene C, Rinchuse D, Stockstill J, editors. TMD and Orthodontics. Cham: Springer; 2015. DOI: 10.1007/978-3-319-19782-1_7

[6] Chigurupati R, Mehra P. Surgical management of idiopathic condylar resorption: Orthognathic surgery versus temporomandibular total joint replacement. Oral and Maxillofacial Surgery Clinics of North America. 2018;**30**(3):355-367, ISSN 1042-3699, ISBN 9780323614047. DOI: 10.1016/j.coms.2018.05.004

[7] Mercuri LG, Edibam NR, Giobbie-Hurder A. Fourteen-year follow-up of a patient-fitted total temporomandibular joint reconstruction system. Journal of Oral and Maxillofacial Surgery. 2007;**65**(6):1140-1148

[8] Wolford LM, Cardenas L. Idiopathic condylar resorption: Diagnosis, treatment protocol and outcomes. American Journal of Orthodontics and Dentofacial Orthopedics. 1999;**116**:667-677

[9] Alsabban L, Amarista FJ, Mercuri LG, Perez D. Idiopathic condylar resorption: A survey and review of the literature. Journal of Oral and Maxillofacial Surgery. 2018;**76**(11):2316.e1-2316.e13. DOI: 10.1016/j.joms.2018.07.008 Epub 2018 Jul 19

[10] Valladares-Neto J, Acioli GMR, Teodoro AB, Evangelista K, Furquim BD', MAG S. Conservative and minimally invasive approaches to control idiopathic condylar resorption: A scoping review. International Journal of Oral and Maxillofacial Surgery. 2023;**52**(11):1188-1196. DOI: 10.1016/j.ijom.2023.05.003 Epub 2023

[11] Arnett GW, Gunson MJ. Risk factors in the initiation of condylar resorption. Seminars in Orthodontics. 2013;**19**:81-88. DOI: 10.1053/j.sodo.2012.11.001

[12] Wolford LM, Galiano A. Adolescent internal condylar resorption (AICR) of the temporomandibular joint, part 1: A review for diagnosis and treatment considerations. Cranio. 2019;**37**:35-44. DOI: 10.1080/08869634.2017.1386752

[13] Posnick JC, Kaban LB, Alimanovic D, Pedersen TK, Matzen LH, Stoustrup P.

Comparing clinical and radiological manifestations of adolescent idiopathic condylar resorption and juvenile idiopathic arthritis in the temporomandibular joint. Journal of Oral and Maxillofacial Surgery. 2021. J Oral Maxillofac Surg. 2021 Sep;79(9):1809.;**79**(4):774-785. DOI: 10.1016/j.joms.2021.04.025 Epub 2021 Jun 4

[14] He Y, Lin H, Lin Q, Lu L, Li M, Li Q, et al. Morphologic changes in idiopathic condylar resorption with different degrees of bone loss. Oral Surgery, Oral Medicine, Oral Pathology, Oral Radiology. 2019;**128**(3):332-340. DOI: 10.1016/j.0000.2019.05.013 Epub 2019 Jun 6

[15] Arnett GW, Milam SB, Gottesman L. Progressive mandibular retrusion–idiopathic condylar resorption. Part I. American Journal of Orthodontics and Dentofacial Orthopedics. 1996;**110**(1):8-15

[16] Arnett GW, Milam SB, Gottesman L. Progressive mandibular retrusion-idiopathic condylar resorption. Part II. American Journal of Orthodontics and Dentofacial Orthopedics. 1996;**110**(2):117-127

[17] Scheerlink JPO, Stoelinga PJW, Blijdorp PA, et al. Sagittal split advancement osteotomies stabilized with miniplates: 2-5 years follow-up. International Journal of Oral and Maxillofacial Surgery. 1994;**23**:127-131

[18] Wolford LM. Idiopathic condylar resorption of the temporomandibular joint in teenage girls (cheer-leaders syndrome). Proceedings (Baylor University. Medical Center). 2001;**14**(3):246-252

[19] Gunson MJ, Arnett GW. Pathophysiology and pharmacologic control of osseous mandibular condylar resorption. The Journal of Maxillofacial and Oral Surgery. 2013;**71**(1):4

[20] Tanimoto K, Awada T, Onishi A, Kubo N, Asakawa Y, Kunimatsu R, et al. Characteristics of the maxillofacial morphology in patients with idiopathic mandibular condylar resorption. Journal of Clinical Medicine. 2022;**11**(4):952. DOI: 10.3390/jcm11040952

[21] Gunson MJ, Arnett GW, Formby B, et al. Oral contraceptive pill use and abnormal menstrual cycles in women with severe condylar resorption: A case for low serum 17 beta-estradiol as a major factor in progressive condylar resorption. American Journal of Orthodontics and Dentofacial Orthopedics. 2009;**136**:772-779

[22] Milam SB. TMJ osteoarthritis. In: Laskin DM, Greene CS, Hylander WL, editors. Tempomandibular Disorders: An Evidence-Based Approach to Diagnosis and Treatment. Chicago: Quintessence; 2006. pp. 105-123

[23] Yuan M, Xie Q, Shen P, Yang C. Do sex hormone imbalances contribute to idiopathic condylar resorption? International Journal of Oral and Maxillofacial Surgery. 2021;**50**(9):1244-1248. DOI: 10.1016/j.ijom.2021.01.017 Epub 2021 Feb 23

[24] Hoppenreijs TJ. Evaluation of condylar resorption before and after orthognathic surgery. Seminars in Orthodontics. 2013;**19**(2):106-115

[25] Hoppenreijs TJM, Freihofer HPM, Stoelinga PJW, et al. Condylar remodeling after LeFort I and bimaxillary osteotomies in patients with anterior open bite. A clinical and radiological study. International Journal of Oral and Maxillofacial Surgery. 1998;**27**:81-91

[26] Borstlap WA, Stoelinga PJ, Hoppenreijs TJ, et al. Stabilisation of sagittal split advancement osteotomies with miniplates: A prospective, multicentre study with two-year follow-up. Part III–condylar remodelling and resorption. International Journal of Oral and Maxillofacial Surgery. 2004;**33**(7):649-655

[27] de Leeuw R, Boering G, Stegenga B, et al. Radiographic signs of temporomandibular joint osteoarthrosis and internal derangement 30 years after nonsurgical treatment. Oral Surgery, Oral Medicine, Oral Pathology, Oral Radiology, and Endodontics. 1995;**79**(3):382-392

[28] Nogami S, Yamauchi K, Odashima K, Ito K, Iikubo M, Kumasaka A, et al. Influence of oestrogen deficiency and excessive mechanical stress on condylar head of mandible. Oral Diseases. 2020;**26**(8):1718-1726. DOI: 10.1111/odi.13452 Epub 2020 Jul 15

[29] Wolford LM, Mercuri LG, Schneiderman ED, et al. Twenty-year follow-up study on a patient-fitted temporomandibular joint prosthesis: The techmedica/TMJ concepts device. Journal of Oral and Maxillofacial Surgery. 2015;**73**(5):952-960

[30] Coleta KE, Wolford LM, Gon¸calves JR, et al. Maxillo-mandibular counter-clockwise rotation and mandibular advancement with TMJ concepts total joint prostheses: Part II–airway changes and stability. International Journal of Oral and Maxillofacial Surgery. 2009;**38**(3):228-235

[31] Alimanovic D, Pedersen TK, Matzen LH, Stoustrup P. Comparing clinical and radiological manifestations of adolescent idiopathic condylar resorption and juvenile idiopathic arthritis in the temporomandibular joint. Journal of Oral and Maxillofacial Surgery. 2021;**79**(4):774-785. DOI: 10.1016/j.joms.2020.10.032 Epub 2020 Oct 23

[32] Posnick JC, Kaban LB. A conceptual framework for treating jaw deformities in patients with abnormal condyles: Preservation versus replacement of the glenoid fossa-disc-condyle-ramus. International Journal of Oral and Maxillofacial Surgery. 2022;**51**(1):98-103. DOI: 10.1016/j.ijom.2021.03.010 Epub 2021 Apr 10

[33] Wolford LM, Kesterke MJ, Craig E, Harrison CEI. The efficacy of patient-fitted total joint prostheses and orthognathic surgery to reconstruct patients with congenital craniofacial deformities and temporomandibular joint malformation: A systematic review. Frontiers of Oral and Maxillofacial Medicine. 2023;**5**:21

[34] Mercuri LG, Handelman CS. Idiopathic condylar resorption: What should we do? Oral and Maxillofacial Surgery Clinics of North America. 2020;**32**(1):105-116. DOI: 10.1016/j.coms.2019.09.001 Epub 2019 Nov 1

[35] Zuleima C, Breton P, Bouletreau P. Management of dentoskeletal deformity due to condylar resorption: Literature review. Oral Surgery, Oral Medicine, Oral Pathology, Oral Radiology. 2016;**121**(2):126-132

Chapter 6

Active Condylar Hyperplasia: An Evaluation of Surgical Therapy

Vladimír Machoň and Daniela Chroustová

Abstract

Condylar hyperplasia (CH) is a postnatal growth abnormality characterized by facial asymmetry and malocclusion and results from excessive growth of the articular process of the mandible. Histologically, CH is characterized by hypertrophic cartilage of the articular head with the presence of cartilaginous islands in the subchondral portion of the head. Depending on the growth activity, condylar hyperplasia is divided into active form (continued growth resulting in worsening asymmetry) and passive form (pathological growth is terminated, asymmetry no longer worsens, and the condition remains stable). Treatment depends on the form of CH activity. In the active form, treatment aims to stop the pathological growth. This is achieved by condylar shaving, where 3 mm to 5 mm of cartilage is removed from the top of the articular head. In most cases, orthodontic treatment is required, possibly with definitive correction through orthognathic surgery. In the case of the passive form (when growth activity is not confirmed), orthodontic therapy and surgery are used. The authors present a set of 115 patients with active CH in whom growth was surgically arrested. Of the postoperative complications, postoperative disc dislocation was the most common (7.8%). Surgical therapy for active condylar hyperplasia is fully effective, with minimal complications.

Keywords: temporomandibular joint, condylar hyperplasia, surgery, complications, condylectomy

1. Introduction

Condylar hyperplasia (CH) is a postnatal growth abnormality characterized by facial asymmetry and malocclusion and results from excessive growth of the articular process of the mandible [1, 2].

This abnormality was first described by Robert Adams in 1836 [1, 3].

This disorder arises due to accelerated growth activity in adolescents or prolonged growth activity in adult patients. It is most common between the ages of 10 and 30, with a higher incidence of CH in females than in males [3–5].

The exact etiology is unclear, but genetic and hormonal disorders, vascular anomalies, trauma and tumors are all considered to contribute. It may involve a response to condylar overload or to a present infection [1, 6, 7].

Histologically, CH is characterized by hypertrophic cartilage of the articular head with the presence of cartilaginous islands in the subchondral portion of the head [8–10].

Clinically, condylar hyperplasia is expressed by asymmetry of the face—a shift of the chin towards the contralateral side and an enlarged mandibular body and branch. Intraorally, malocclusion in the sense of an open or crossed bite can be noted. Changes in the mandible may cause alterations in the alveolus of the maxilla, resulting in changes in the canting of the occlusal plane. The temporomandibular joint (TMJ) clinically shows no signs of pain, TMJ movement is unrestricted, and no auditory phenomena are present [1].

A number of divisions can be used for CH classification.

In 1986 [11], Obwegeser and Makek classified condylar hyperplasia into three groups according to the type of growth:

1. hemimandibular hyperplasia (three-dimensional enlargement of one side of the mandible, including enlargement of the condyle, the condylar neck and the ascending and horizontal ramus) (**Figure 1a**);

2. hemimandibular elongation (elongation of the condylar process associated with displacement of the mandible and chin to the unaffected side in the horizontal plane) (**Figure 1b**);

3. mixed form.

Wolford [12] classifies condylar hyperplasia into four groups according to the histological origin of the hyperplasia:

Type 1—characterized by accelerated growth of the condylar process, which may be unilateral (type 1B) or bilateral (type 1A, leading to prognation);

Type 2—enlargement of the articular process due to osteochondroma of the articular head. There is a distinction between type 2A, where the osteochondroma is endophytic, and type 2B, where the osteochondroma of the articular head is exophytic;

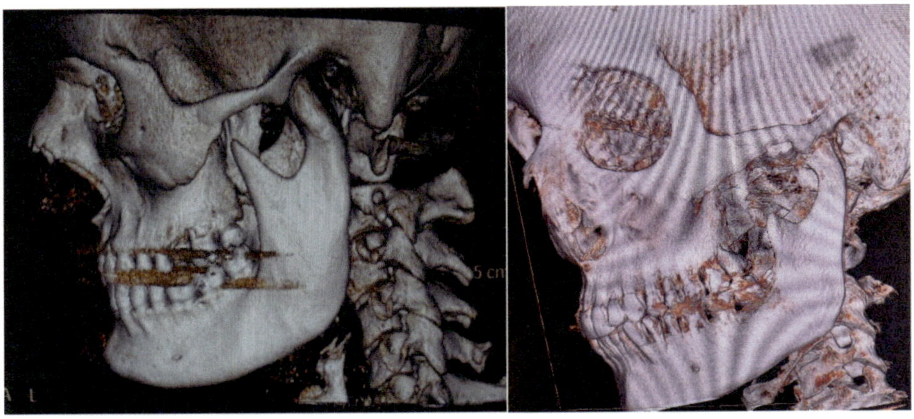

Figure 1.
(a) Hemimandibular hyperplasia. (b) Hemimandibular elongation.

Type 3—condylar hyperplasia due to other benign tumors;

Type 4—condylar hyperplasia due to malignant tumors of the articular processes.

Depending on the direction of excessive growth, clinical manifestation can be divided into two groups [1]:

a. vertical form (dominated by growth in condylar length)—clinically characterized by an open bite with a shift of the mandibular angle and elongation of the mandibular branch on the affected side, with a deviation of the middle of the chin to the affected side;

b. rotational form (dominated by growth in condylar width)—clinically characterized by crossbite and a shift of the mandibular centre and incisor point to the unaffected side.

Depending on the growth activity, according to Laskin [1] condylar hyperplasia is divided into:

Active—continued growth resulting in worsening asymmetry;

Passive—pathological growth is terminated, asymmetry no longer worsens, and the condition remains stable (**Figures 2–5**).

1.1 CH diagnosis

The diagnosis of CH is based on a combination of clinical symptoms and imaging methods; however, only histological examination will provide a definitive diagnosis [13].

X-ray and CT (possibly CBCT) provide information on the type of asymmetry, shape and size of the articular process, and mandibular branch and body [13, 14]. To determine the therapeutic approach, it is necessary not only to make a diagnosis of CH but also to determine whether the CH exhibits positive or negative growth activity. This determination can be made by comparing bite ratios or facial asymmetry over time (comparing radiographs and bite patterns). Nonetheless, this is only an orthodontic evaluation, and to determine whether growth activity is continuing

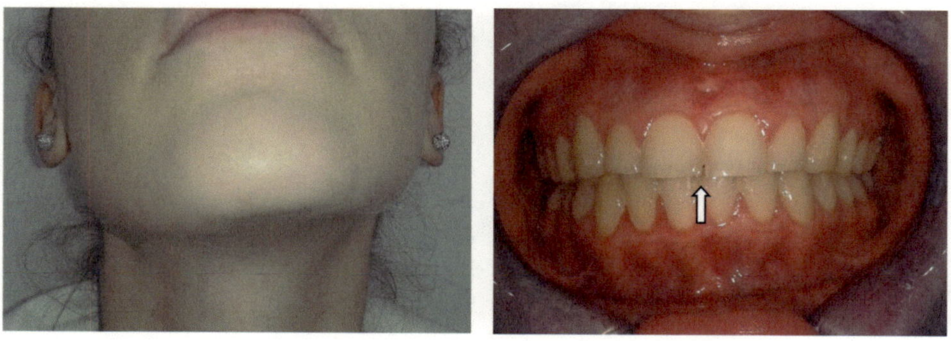

Figure 2.
(a) A 24-year-old female patient. (b) Hemimandibular hyperplasia—clinical view. Enlargement and elongation of the affected half of the mandibular body, mandibular branch, and articular process. The image in (b) shows occlusion, while the arrow indicates the centre of the lower dental arch.

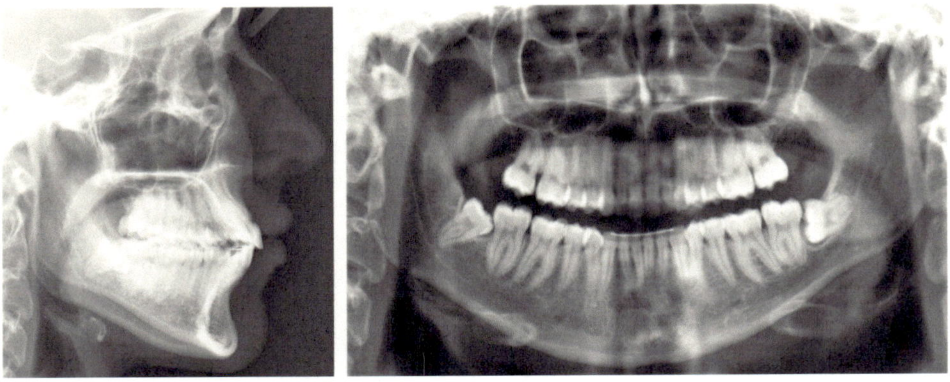

Figure 3.
(a) A 24-year-old female patient. (b) Hemimandibular hyperplasia—tele X-ray and panoramic image.

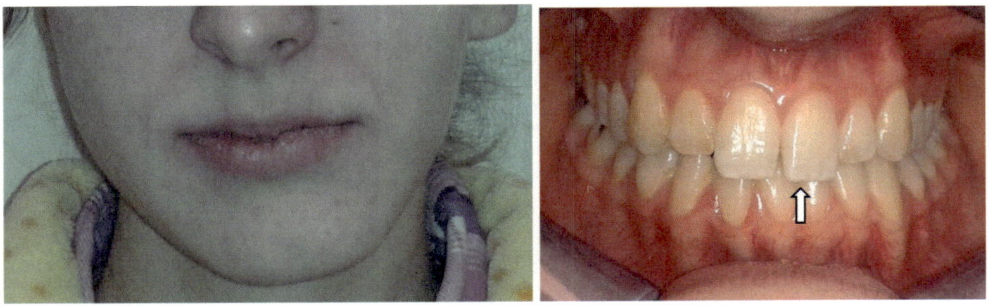

Figure 4.
(a) An 18-year-old female patient. (b) Hemimandibular elongation. Shift of the mandible and chin to the unaffected side in the horizontal plane. The image in (b) shows occlusion, while the arrow indicates the centre of the lower dental arch.

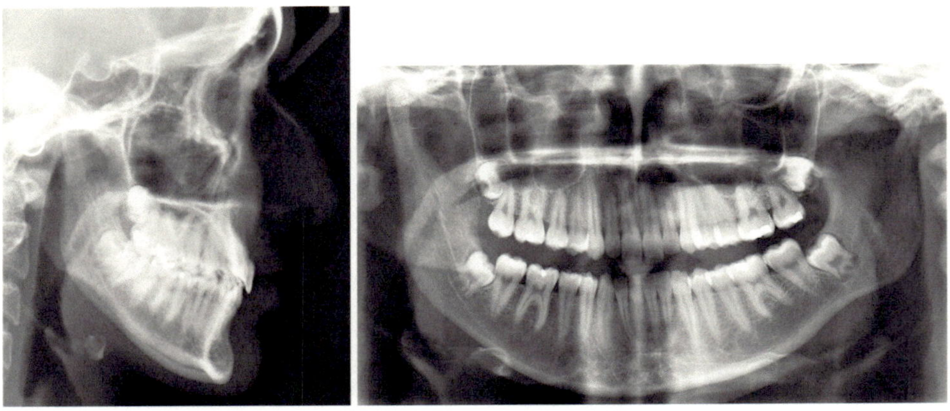

Figure 5.
(a) An 18-year-old female patient. (b) Hemimandibular elongation—tele X-ray and panoramic image.

or has ended, planar skeletal scintigraphy (simple two-dimensional imaging (2D), three-dimensional imaging (3D), single photon emission computed tomography (SPECT), or a combination of SPECT/CT) are used. These methods use the affinity of intravenously administered technetium-99 m for skeletal osteoblastic activity.

If growth activity is positive, the distribution of technetium in the affected condyle will be at least 10% higher than in the unaffected condyle [14].

Boos-Lima [15] evaluated these three methods in his review, highlighting SPECT/CT as the most accurate, but the differences in sensitivity and specificity between the methods were not significant.

1.2 Therapy

Treatment depends on the form of CH activity.

In the active form (with confirmed growth activity), treatment aims to stop the pathological growth. This is achieved by condylar shaving, where 3–5 mm of cartilage is removed from the top of the articular head together with the subchondral bone [16]. In the case of significant elongation with extension of the pathologically altered articular process, a high condylectomy (where a larger part of or the entire articular head is removed) can be used. Better skeletal symmetry is ultimately achieved by

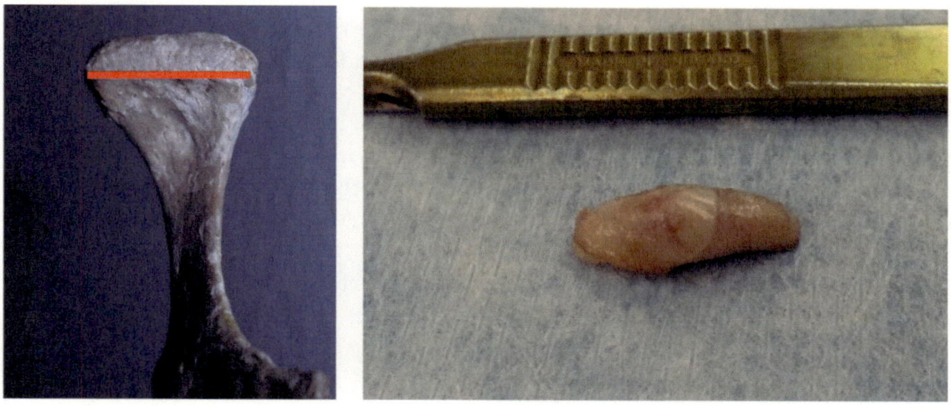

Figure 6.
Condylar shaving.

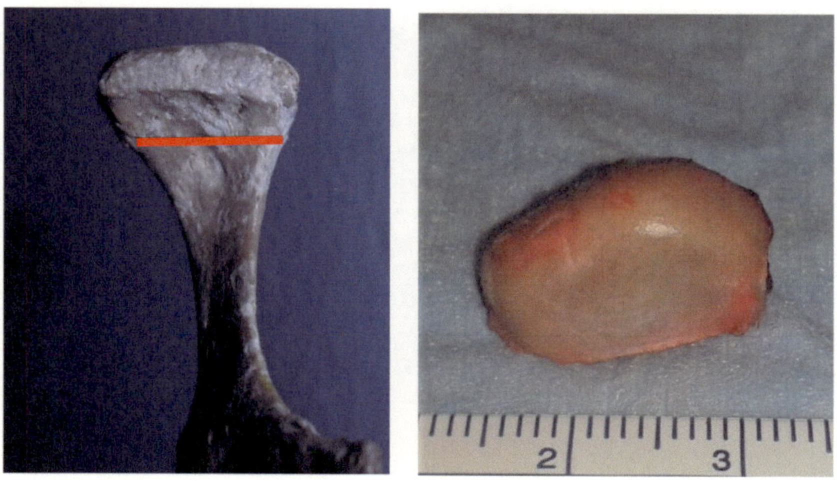

Figure 7.
High condylectomy.

removing the difference in size between the affected and unaffected condyle. In most cases, orthodontic treatment is required, possibly with definitive correction through orthognathic surgery [17].

In the case of the passive form (when growth activity is not confirmed), orthodontic therapy and orthognatic surgery are used (**Figures 6** and 7) [16].

2. Performing surgery for active CH

The basic surgical approach to condylar shaving is the external one—preauricular or endaural. In the preauricular approach, the incision is made in front of the auricle, whereas in the endaural approach, the incision is made in the upper front part of the auricle (the same as with the preauricular approach) but then passes to the edge of the tragus cartilage. In both cases, the deep layer of the temporal fascia is penetrated, and the zygomatic arch and the joint capsule become evident in this layer [5, 16].

Compared to a preauricular incision, the endaural incision is more esthetic, and the scar is less visible [16].

The main risks of this surgical approach are injury to the facial or auriculotemporal nerve, injury to the superficial temporal vein and artery, perforation of the ear canal, and necrosis of the tragus cartilage [16].

The cut to open the joint capsule is made using a vertical incision, and in the upper part, the cut is supplemented with a horizontal incision of several millimeters. The resulting incision of the joint capsule then resembles the letter 'T'. After freeing the lateral attachment of the disc, an elevator is used to make the articular head clearly visible [16].

Condylar shaving and high condylectomies are performed with a piezo saw to minimize the risk of injury to the soft tissue structures around the joint [18].

Another approach mentioned for condylar shaving and condylectomy is the intraoral one, where a retromolar incision is made [19, 20]. This incision is associated with limited visualization. However, compared to the external approaches, it minimizes

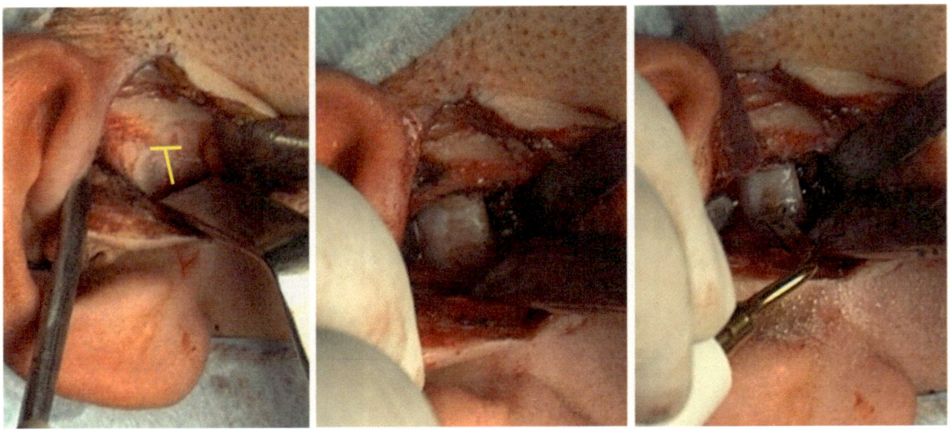

Figure 8.
(a) A view of the joint capsule with a 'T' incision. In (b), the articular process and the head are visible. The image in (c) shows a condylectomy performed using piezosurgery, in this case a high condylectomy. The anterior and posterior margins of the articular process are protected by elevator or possibly Dunn-Dautrey temporomandibular joint condyle retractors.

nerve damage in the TMJ area and is not associated with esthetic drawbacks from postoperative scarring (**Figures 8–10**) [19, 20].

It is very important to limit trauma to the disc and not disturb its integrity. Preserving the disc will ensure the full functionality of the joint. The disc should be checked at the end of the procedure. It can be left loose, without its position being adjusted [3, 21]. Cascone [22] recommends fixing the *ligamentum laterale* and the disc to the lateral part of the articular process. This restores the anatomical traction of the disc to the articular process structure. This fixation is performed with sutures fixed to an anchor inserted into the articular process.

Pathological growth activity is fully stopped by condylar shaving, while facial symmetry is ensured by subsequent orthodontic or orthodontic-surgical therapy [5]. However, proportional condylectomy is used to improve postoperative symmetry

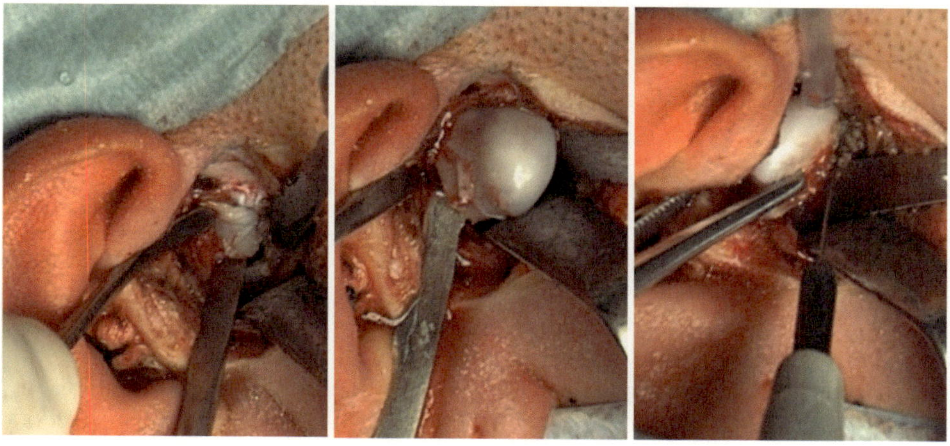

Figure 9.
(a) The condylectomy utilizes an elevator, which gently extrudes the articular head laterally as shown in (b). (c) The head is gently grasped with forceps, and the lateral pterygoid muscle tendon is released with electrocautery.

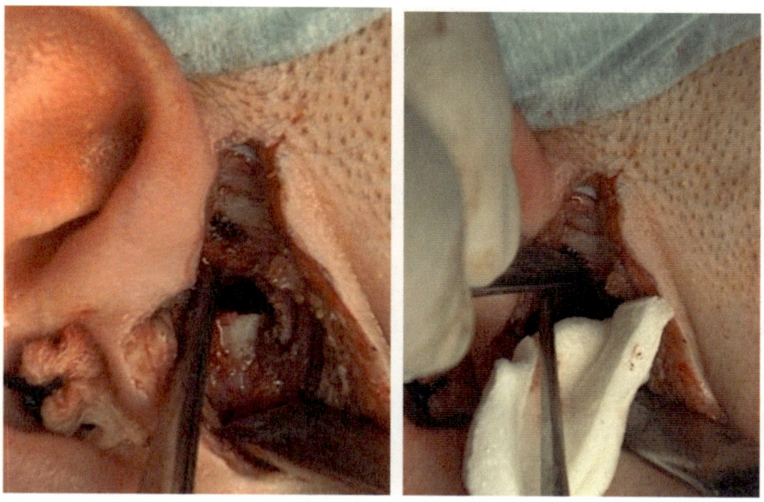

Figure 10.
(a) View of the lower joint space after a high condylectomy. (b) Inspection of the inferior disc surface is followed by the insertion of haemostatic foam into the surgical wound. This is followed by wound closure.

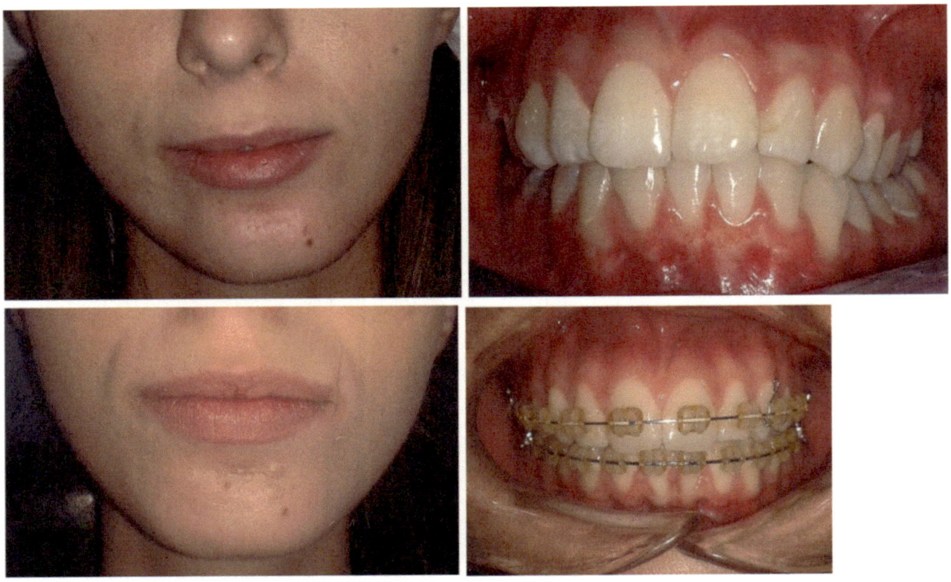

Figure 11.
A 14-year-old female patient with hemimandibular elongation. She was indicted for a proportional high condylectomy. (a, b) show apparent mandibular asymmetry and an asymmetrical bite. (c, d) show the patient 2 years after surgery, in the final stages of orthodontic therapy.

and reduce the need for facial asymmetry correction by orthognathic surgery. This consists of virtual planning, whereby a bilateral comparison of the mandibular ramus is made to determine the difference in the height of the rounded articular processes. This difference then determines how much the affected (growing articular process) is to be shortened [5, 20–22]. To ensure an accurate condylectomy, cutting guides are 3D printed and positioned in the sigmoid notch (Haas) or fixed to the lateral surface of the articular head [5, 22].

An alternative method to condylar shaving and high condylectomy was published by Hashemi [19], who removed the growth zone of the condyle by coagulation mode cauterization (three phases of 5 seconds duration with a voltage of 65 mV). The electrocautery probe was introduced into the condyle after drilling, from an intraoral approach.

The ideal time for surgical treatment is after skeletal growth has stopped. In paediatric patients, with a growing skeleton, it is advisable to wait until the surgical solution of active CH, and to dispensary the patient. The author performs control scintigraphy in these patients after a year [16]. At the time of the expected termination of skeletal growth, it is advisable to proceed to surgical therapy in case of significant asymmetries. Continued growth activity on the non-operated side can compensate for the asymmetry (**Figure 11a–d**) [16, 21].

3. Postoperative care

Postoperative care consists of rehabilitating the mouth opening. The patient starts on the 1st postoperative day, when they spontaneously open their mouth as far as pain permits. If the mouth opening is altered, physiotherapy is used, where the patient practices opening their mouth under the supervision of a physiotherapist [16]. Sembronio [5] recommends early mouth-opening physiotherapy so that normal mouth opening is achieved within 10 days. In the event facial nerve function is altered, facial nerve function rehabilitation is begun on the 1st postoperative day. Soft food is recommended for the first 3 days [16]. After surgery, early orthodontic therapy is initiated, and elastic traction is often used to compensate for malocclusion [5, 21]. It is important to note that the mandible shifts after condylar shaving and condylectomy, inducing premature contact on the operated side, while the bite opens on the contralateral side. Elastic traction reduces intrusive forces on the operated side. However, it is advisable to fix the traction behind anchoring elements used in orthodontics (screws, mini-splints), thereby minimizing unwanted tooth extrusion and balancing occlusion [23].

4. Own experience, complications in assessing surgical therapy

Between 2013 and 2022, 725 patients were diagnosed with facial asymmetry due to enlargement of the articular process of the mandibular branch at the Department of Oral Maxillofacial Surgery at Charles University and Faculty Hospital Prague. In all these patients, tumor lesion of the condyle was excluded by panoramic X-ray and CT (CBCT). The cohort consisted of 490 females (67%) and 235 males (33%), with a mean age of 22.2 years. In all these patients, scintigraphy was performed to assess the presence of pathological growth activity (intravenous administration of the radiopharmaceutical technician. If activity was confirmed, the distribution of technicium in the affected condyle was at least 10% higher than in the unaffected condyle).

In 606 patients (407 women and 199 men, with a mean age of 22 years), pathological growth activity was not demonstrated by scintigraphy, and these patients underwent planned orthodontic and orthodontic-surgical therapy.

In 119 patients (16.4%), namely, 83 women (69%) and 36 men (31%) with a mean age of 22.7 years, one-sided growth activity was demonstrated by scintigraphy. Surgical management (condylar shaving, high condylectomy) was recommended for these patients. One hundred fifteen patients accepted this approach (96.6%), while four patients refused the proposed surgery (3.4%).

All 115 patients who underwent surgical treatment were histologically diagnosed with condylar hyperplasia. The Obwegesser and Makek [11] classification was used to classify CH. Twenty-three patients (20%) had hemimandibular hyperplasia; hemimandibular elongation was observed in 72 patients (63%), while the mixed form was seen in 20 patients (17%).

Of the surgical methods, condylar shaving was used in 94 patients (81%), and 21 patients (19%) underwent proportional high condylectomy.

TMJ function. The mean maximal mouth interincisal opening (MIO) before surgery was 44.6 mm. One year after surgery, the mean MIO was 43.8 mm (all patients had a minimum MIO of 35 mm).

The scarring was rated as satisfactory by the surgeon and patient in all the cases.

Follow-up treatment: eight patients (7%) underwent only condylar shaving without the need for any follow-up treatment, while the bite and facial symmetry were spontaneously corrected to a satisfactory state for the patient. In 78 patients (67%), the bite and facial symmetry were addressed with subsequent orthodontic therapy. In 29 patients (26%), follow-up therapy included not only orthodontic treatment but also orthognathic surgery (**Figure 12**).

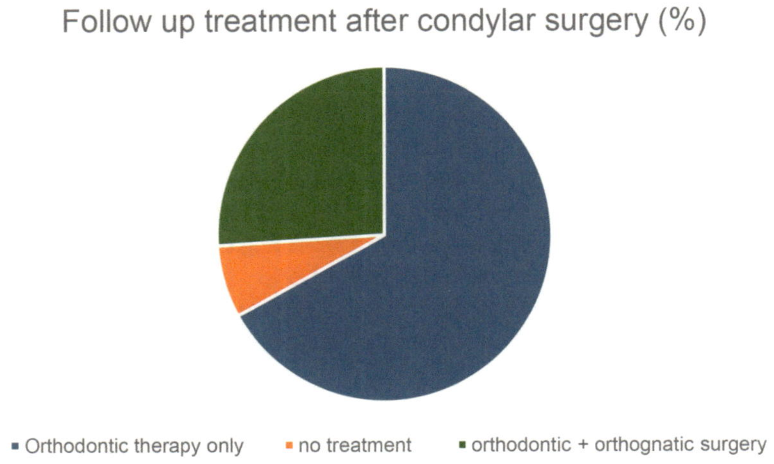

Figure 12.
Follow-up treatment.

4.1 Complications

All patients in the cohort were followed up regularly for at least 1 year.

Facial nerve injury was noted in three patients (2.6%). In all three cases, this was a frontal branch injury and only a temporary disability (full recovery of function occurred within 1, 2 and 6 months). The complications were managed with physiotherapy.

Auriculotemporal nerve injury occurred in two patients (1.7%), and in both cases was only a temporary disability (full recovery of function occurred within 6 and 12 months). The complications were managed with long-term vitamin therapy.

Inflammatory complications were present in one case (female, 22 years old), who experienced swelling of the outer side of the auricle with redness and pain on the third day after surgery. This was cartilage inflammation of the auricle, *perichodritis auriculae*. The condition was managed with an incision, irrigation and antibiotic therapy for 7 days. Currently, 6 years after the inflammatory complication, the auricle is without signs of deformity and the joint is fully functional (**Figure 13**).

TMJ dysfunction was noted in a total of nine patients (7.8%) after surgery. All the cases involved disc dislocation (confirmed by TMJ ultrasound). In four patients, clinical manifestations presented as painless joint locking, which patients started to notice during the 1st month after surgery. In four patients, clinical manifestations of TMJ dysfunction presented as painless regular peeling (two patients developed auditory phenomena during the first month after surgery, and the other two patients between the third and sixth month).

All patients with disc dislocation and repositioning started conservative therapy (home physiotherapy). Two patients improved within 1 month, while six patients (5.2%) could not eliminate the auditory phenomena.

In one case, a closed lock (due to anterior disc dislocation without repositioning) was noted up to 12 months after condylar shaving.

Pain was noted in six patients (5.2%), and in all cases, was myogenic discomfort localized to the masseter muscle. Pain was observed in all patients between one and 3 months after surgery. In three cases, this was muscle pain on the operated side and in three cases on the contralateral side. The condition was alleviated for all the patients by physiotherapy. TMJ pain was not recorded (**Figure 14**).

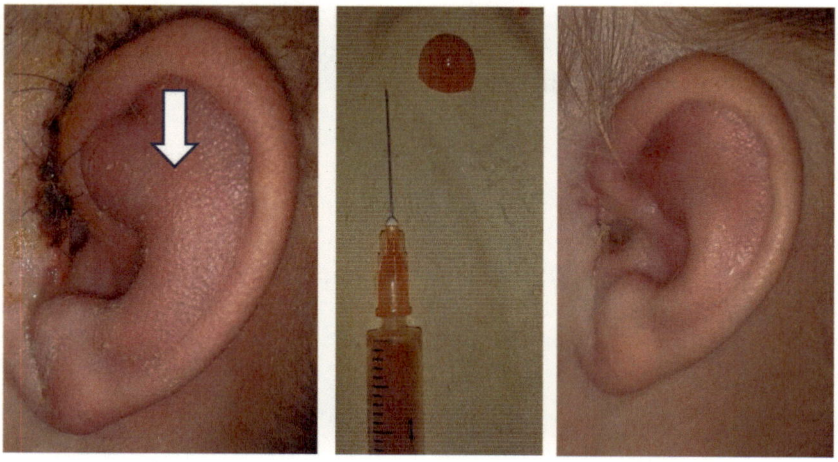

Figure 13.
Clinical photo of a patient with inflammatory complication of the auricle, with an inflammatory sample aspirated from the auricle in (b) and the condition 2 weeks later in (c).

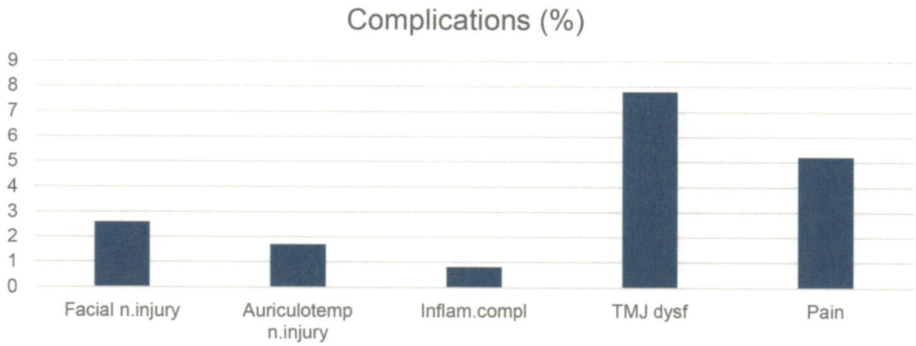

Figure 14.
Complication after condylar shaving, condylectomy.

The results of this cohort are consistent with the results of other authors [5, 21, 22]. Condylar shaving and condylectomy do not imply functional limitation for the joint [5, 21], while pain in the operated joint is not reported [5]. Condylar shaving and condylectomy are surgical methods with minimal complications. The most common complication in the present cohort was TMJ dysfunction in the sense of disc dislocation (7.8%), which persisted in 5.8% of patients 1 year after surgery. Cascone [22] emphasizes the fixation of the disc to the condyle, thereby adjusting the physiological position of the disc.

In contrast, Nitzan [21] emphasizes postoperative therapy, which consists of the distraction of the condyle from direct contact with the disc on the operated side (by elastic traction on the contralateral side). The authors left the disc completely free, without fixation, which could explain the presence of disc dislocation in the postoperative period—it may be the cause of these complications. Among the other complications, muscle pain was the predominant episodic symptom, occurring due to the change in the position of the mandible and, thus, a change in muscle tension. Nonetheless, Saridin [10] reports that there is no difference in disc dislocation and myogenic pain in patients with CH in whom condylectomy was indicated compared with patients without

CH. Limitation of facial nerve function occurred in 2.6% of those operated on, and the limitation was only temporary. This figure is comparable with other authors [3, 5]. Inflammatory complications in the auricle region are indeed rare.

5. Conclusion

Surgical therapy for active condylar hyperplasia is fully effective, with minimal complications. A clear trend is a preference for proportional high condylectomy, which, with early orthodontic therapy, minimizes the need for correction of facial asymmetry through orthognathic surgery.

Author details

Vladimír Machoň[1*] and Daniela Chroustová[2]

1 Faculty Hospital Prague, Department of Oral Maxillofacial Surgery, Charles University, Prague, Czech Republic

2 Faculty Hospital Prague, Department of Nuclear Medicine, Charles University, Prague, Czech Republic

*Address all correspondence to: machonv@seznam.cz

References

[1] Laskin DM, Greene CS, Hylander WL. TMDs. An Evidence-Based Approach to Diagnosis and Treatment. Chicago, IL: Quintessence Publishing; 2006. 548 p

[2] Sun R, Sun L, Sun Z, Li G, Zhao Y, Ma X, et al. A three-dimensional study of hemimandibular hyperplasia, hemimandibular elongation, solitary condylar hyperplasia, simple mandibular asymmetry and condylar osteoma or osteochondroma. Journal of Cranio-Maxillo-Facial Surgery. 2019;**47**:1665e1675

[3] Turvey TA, Hannan E, Brader T, Bhatt P, Oliverson T, Magraw CBL, et al. Active unilateral condylar hyperplasia treated with simultaneous condylectomy and orthognathic surgery: A clinical report. Journal of Oral and Maxillofacial Surgery. 2022;**80**:1593-1612

[4] Raijmakers PG, Karssemakers LH, Tuinzing DB. Female predominance and effect of gender on unilateral condylar hyperplasia: A review and meta-analysis. Journal of Oral and Maxillofacial Surgery. 2012;**70**(1):e72-e76

[5] Sembronio S, Tel A, Costa F, Robiony M. An updated protocol for the treatment of condylar hyperplasia: Computer guided proportional condylectomy. Journal of Oral and Maxillofacial Surgery. 2019;**77**:1457-1465

[6] Eduardo AL, Joseph Z, Sean P. Condylar hyperplasia: An updated review of the literature. The Korean Journal of Orthodontics. 2015;**45**:333e340

[7] Olate S, Netto HD, Rodriguezchessa J, Alister JP, De Albergaria BJ, De Moraes M. Mandible condylar hyperplasia: A review of diagnosis and treatment protocol. International Journal of Clinical and Experimental Medicine. 2013;**6**(9):727-737

[8] Karssemakers LHE, Nolte JW, Tuinzing DB, GEJ L, Becking AG, Raijmakers OG. Impact of bone volume upon condylar activity in patients with unilateral condylar hyperplasia. Journal of Oral and Maxillofacial Surgery. 2018;**76**(10):2177-2182

[9] Machoň V, Bartoš M, Suchý T, Levorová J, Foltán R. Micro-computed tomography evaluation of bone architecture in various forms of unilateral condylar hyperplasia. International Journal of Oral and Maxillofacial Surgery. 2023;**52**(1):44-50

[10] Saridin CP, Raijmakers PG, Slootweg PJ, Tuinzing DB, Becking AG, van der Waal I. Unilateral condylar hyperactivity: A histopathologic analysis of 47 patients. Journal of Oral and Maxillofacial Surgery. 2010;**68**:47-53

[11] Obwegeser HL, Makek MS. Hemimandibularhyperplasiahemimandibular elongation. Journal of Maxillofacial Surgery. 1986;**14**(4):183-208

[12] Wolford LM, Movahed R, Perez DE. A classification system for conditions causing condylar hyperplasia. Journal of Oral and Maxillofacial Surgery. 2014;**72**(3):567-595

[13] Espinosa S, Covarrubias E, Díaz R, Díaz KT, Cafferata EA. Histologic findings and related diagnostic methods in condylar hyperactivity. International Journal of Oral and Maxillofacial Surgery. 2021;**50**(54-63):17

[14] Karssemakers LHE, Nolte JW, Rehmann C, Raijmakers PG, Becking AG. Diagnostic performance

of SPECT–CT imaging in unilateral condylar hyperplasia. International Journal of Oral and Maxillofacial Surgery. 2023;**52**:199-204

[15] Boos-Lima FBDJ, Guastaldi FPS, Kaban LB, Peacock ZS. Accuracy of skeletal scintigraphy for the evaluation of mandibular growth disorders: A systematic review. International Journal of Oral and Maxillofacial Surgery. 2023;**28**:911-916

[16] Machoň V. Manual of TMJ Surgery; the Prague Approach. Praha: Business Media Praha; 2017. 135 pp

[17] Lippold C, Kruse-Loster B, Danesh G, Joos U, Meyer U. Treatment of hemimandibular hyperplasia: The biological basis of condylectomy. British Journal of Oral and Maxillofacial Surgery. 2007;**45**:353-360

[18] Cascone P, Runci Anastasi R, Maffia F, Vellone V. Slice functional condylectomy and piezosurgery: A proposal in unilateral condylar hyperplasia treatment. The Journal of Craniofacial Surgery. 2021;**32**(5):1836-1837

[19] Hashemi HM, Amirzargar R. Can electrocautery of the mandibular condyle effectively treat condylar hyperplasia? Journal of Cranio-Maxillo-Facial Surgery. 2022;**50**:785e789

[20] Haas OL Jr, Farin˜a R, Herna'ndez-Alfaro F, de Oliveira RB. Minimally invasive intraoral proportional condylectomy with a three-dimensionally printed cutting guide. International Journal of Oral and Maxillofacial Surgery. 2020;**49**:1435-1438

[21] Nitzan DW. 'Adaptable condylectomy' for acquired facial asymmetry and malocclusion caused by temporomandibular joint condylar hyperplasia. International Journal of Oral and Maxillofacial Surgery. 2023;**52**(11):1145-1155

[22] Cascone P, D'Alessandro F, Gallo E, Cicero G, Valentino VV. The role of three-dimensional printing technology as an additional tool in unilateral condylar hyperplasia surgical planning. The Journal of Craniofacial Surgery. 2020;**31**(7):e735-e738

[23] Abboud WA, Romano R, Ledermann S, Shashua D, Naddaf R, Tulchinsky M, et al. Can condylectomy alone achieve facial symmetry in patients with hemimandibular hyperplasia (condylar hyperplasia type 2)? The Journal of Craniofacial Surgery. 2020;**31**(7):e735-e738

Chapter 7

Alloplastic Temporomandibular Total Joint Replacement

Ryan J. McCoy and David J. Psutka

Abstract

Alloplastic temporomandibular total joint reconstruction provides an effective surgical treatment option for patients with end-stage temporomandibular joint disease. While temporomandibular disorders are often initially managed with non-surgical modalities, severe ankylosis, aberrant anatomic deformity, or loss of primary function necessitates surgical intervention in patients with late-stage disease. Modern advancements in the field of temporomandibular joint replacement, especially over the last three to four decades, have improved upon initial challenges of poor prosthetic design and improper material selection. Modern alloplastic prosthetic devices, including both stock and custom patient-fitted prostheses, have been shown to be both safe and effective in restoring temporomandibular form and function. Alloplastic temporomandibular total joint replacement now represents a successful surgical solution with advantages including improved accessibility, reduced operative time, earlier return to mobilization, and lower morbidity risks than autogenous methods. This chapter will provide an overview of the fundamental principles of temporomandibular joint replacement, indications for surgery, patient selection, stock versus custom prostheses, outcomes, and potential complications with reference to the current body of literature.

Keywords: alloplastic, temporomandibular joint, reconstruction, joint replacement, orthopedic, joint, prostheses, custom, stock

1. Introduction

Alloplastic total joint replacement (TJR) has become a safe, widely accepted, and accessible procedure in the treatment of end-stage temporomandibular joint (TMJ) disease [1]. As early as 1840, the fundamental idea of interposing artificial or exogenic materials between diseased joint surfaces was implemented by the American surgeon Dr. John Murray Carnochan, who placed wood between the articular surfaces of an ankylosed mandible after rudimentary gap arthroplasty [1]. Since that time, the field of temporomandibular total joint replacement (TMJ TJR) has had a colorful history filled with numerous attempts to successfully reconstruct the temporomandibular joint using various alloplastic materials. The intricate role of the TMJ in mastication, speech, and airway maintenance presented unique challenges in creating a viable joint replacement device [2]. Initially, TMJ reconstruction was performed only in severe cases of developmental maxillofacial deformity, inflammatory joint disease, ankylosis, or previous tumor resection [2]. As a result, early cases were rare and reporting of long-term complications was limited. Over the span of nearly a half-century, numerous synthetic materials including silicone elastomers, Teflon and Proplast, various acrylics, and other novel substances were utilized in search of the ideal alloplastic material [2]. As alloplastic total joint replacement became increasingly more common, various systems were developed and subsequently discontinued with a large variance in reported success rates, leading patients to require an increasing number of revisions of previous failed reconstructions, thus adding an additional layer of complexity [1–3].

The late 1990s brought about the advent of what is now considered the modern-day alloplastic temporomandibular joint replacement prosthesis. The global oral and maxillofacial surgery community has since made substantial progress in addressing the initial shortcomings that characterized historical alloplastic TMJ reconstruction [4]. Inappropriate prosthetic models, inadequate clinical trial design, and inattention to outcomes outlined in orthopedic literature have been amended with well-designed pre-market trials for both stock and patient-specific TMJ TJR devices [4]. As a result of these improvements, alloplastic total joint replacement now represents a highly effective surgical solution for advanced TMJ dysfunction or ankylosis, greatly benefitting the form and function of patients with late-stage disease.

2. Modern alloplastic TMJ reconstruction

The core principles of total TMJ reconstruction surgery include the resection of significantly degenerated articular structures due to inflammatory arthritic disease, the release of bony or fibrous ankylosis, the return of non-morbid occlusion, the re-establishment of vertical mandibular ramal height, the restoration of articular surfaces, and the creation of barriers to prevent further ankylosis and maintain jaw mobilization [1, 2]. Alloplastic TJR prostheses consist of two components that reconstruct the articulating surfaces of the temporomandibular joint: a mandibular ramal component and a glenoid fossa component. The mandibular component reconstructs the condylar process and a portion of the ramus of the mandible. It is typically fabricated out of titanium (Ti-6AL-4V) alloy and/or nickel-containing cobalt-chromium-molybdenum (Co-Cr-Mo) alloy due to the biocompatibility and strength of these materials. The glenoid fossa component is commonly fabricated out of an ultrahigh molecular weight polyethylene (UHMWPE), with or without an unalloyed titanium mesh backing. These alloplastic components are designed to withstand normal occlusal loads over the full range of motion while prosthetic components are stably fixated [2]. This combination of materials has been found to provide an optimal balance of flexibility, strength, wear and corrosion resistance, and biocompatibility to recreate the complex functions of the TMJ.

2.1 Advantages and disadvantages

The advantages of alloplastic TMJ replacement are numerous. Stock alloplastic systems are widely available and can be inventoried for immediate use as needed [5]. Unlike autogenous TMJ replacement options, alloplastic reconstruction also avoids the donor site morbidity risks associated with tissue harvest. For example, potential complications such as pneumothorax, increased anesthesia time, and post operative abductor weakness of the ipsilateral upper limb seen with costochondral graft harvest can be avoided [5]. The lack of donor site is also beneficial in decreasing surgical time, which is an important advantage where operating room resources are scarce. Patient-specific alloplastic options provide further benefit as they are custom manufactured to conform to each patient's anatomy, decreasing the time needed for implant fitting and anatomic adaptation, as well as implantation. Unlike autogenous grafts, alloplastic implants are also not vulnerable to failure secondary to foreign body reaction from particulate matter from previous failed prostheses, which is a useful advantage in patients requiring revision of prior reconstructions [2]. Lastly, patients who undergo alloplastic TMJ replacement are not limited to delayed physical therapy and can often begin treatment in the immediate post-operative phase.

Although alloplastic TMJ replacement is an effective tool in temporomandibular joint replacement, it is not without disadvantages. There is a notable expense associated with both the computer-aided surgical simulation (CASS) and fabrication of the alloplastic components. Although surgical operating room and anesthesia fees may be less than with autogenous graft harvest and implantation, the fabrication cost of the alloplastic implants can be a significant barrier for many patients or health networks [5]. Another potential disadvantage associated with alloplastic TMJ replacement is longevity. Although the current expected lifespan of alloplastic TMJ TJR devices is not explicitly defined in the literature, recent studies have shown excellent durability of at least 10–20 years for modern TMJ TJR devices [3, 6–9]. However, the need for revision surgery is presently unpredictable as long-term data regarding device longevity is still unknown. Although the biocompatibility of modern alloplastic joint components is well documented, material hypersensitivity remains a concern associated with any alloplastic joint replacement. The rate of aseptic failure due to alloplastic TMJ replacement, although infrequent, is not yet well defined [10]. The rare potential for wear debris and the subsequent biological response also represents a potential complication that cannot be overlooked [2]. Lastly, alloplastic TMJ joint replacement is currently only indicated in skeletally mature individuals which limits suitability in younger patients [2].

2.2 Indications, contraindications, and patient selection

The indications for alloplastic joint replacement are dictated by the fundamental goals and principles of total TMJ reconstruction. The principal objectives of any TMJ reconstructive surgery, be it autogenous or alloplastic, involve the cost-effective enhancement of mandibular form and function with concomitant pain reduction, while also preventing further morbidity [11]. One of the most common indications for alloplastic TMJ reconstruction is late-stage degenerative joint disease secondary to either non-inflammatory or inflammatory arthropathies [2]. Other indications include adolescent internal condylar resorption, recurrent ankylosis, revision of failed alloplastic or autogenous reconstruction, irreparable condylar fracture, avascular necrosis, congenital disorders such as orofacial or oromandibular dysostoses, and neoplasia requiring extensive resection [2, 8, 9]. Relative contraindications for alloplastic TMJ TJR include acute or chronic infection, skeletal immaturity, prosthetic material hypersensitivity, and patients with increased susceptibility to infection secondary to uncontrolled or poorly controlled systemic disease [3].

Patient selection is a critical component of successful total TMJ reconstruction. For skeletally immature patients, autogenous joint replacement or distraction osteogenesis have historically been referred to as the gold-standard methods of TMJ reconstruction [2]. Skeletally mature patients, on the other hand, may benefit from alloplastic joint reconstruction. As more experience is gained with alloplastic TMJ TJR devices, future advancements may allow for the inclusion of patients that have not yet reached skeletal maturity [2]. Mercuri and Swift reported that alloplastic TMJ TJR may also be beneficial in patients whose joints have no potential for continued growth due to severe ankylosis, mutilation, or multiple operations [12]. A stock prosthesis is safe and effective for reconstruction of a non-mutilated joint, however patients who have undergone multiple operations or have significant anatomic mutilation typically require a computer-assisted design/computer-assisted manufactured (CAD/CAM) custom joint prosthesis [2].

It is important to note that dentofacial deformities which require surgical correction frequently exist together with temporomandibular joint disorders. Regardless of whether a patient's TMJ pathology is a causative factor for subsequent dentofacial deformity, or it develops because of a pre-existing jaw deformity, patients with these concomitant conditions may benefit from surgical intervention which includes both alloplastic joint reconstruction and orthognathic surgery [2]. Orthognathic surgeons should realize that healthy and biologically stable temporomandibular joints are necessary for favorable surgical outcomes, with significant TMJ pathology often leading to unsatisfactory results in function, esthetics, pain, and skeletal/occlusal stability. Surgeons must recognize potential TMJ issues in patients with high occlusal plane angle progressively worsening class II morphologies, especially where an anterior open bite exists. Wolford outlines that major surgical advancements in the past 25 years have confirmed that combined temporomandibular joint and orthognathic surgery (C-TJR-OS) can be safely and predictably performed in a single operation with accurate diagnosis and planning (**Figure 1**) [2]. Wolford also notes that in his 25 year experience using patient-fitted TMJ TJR devices, "approximately two-thirds of patients requiring TMJ TJR can benefit from concomitant orthognathic surgery for improvement in function, airway and breathing capabilities, better aesthetic outcomes, and decreased or elimination of pain" [2]. Although an in-depth review of the intricacies of C-TJR-OS is outside the scope of this chapter, it is important to note that typically surgical sequencing involves condylectomy/coronoidectomy, mobilization of the mandible and placement of an intermediate splint, placement of the total joint prostheses, followed by maxillary osteotomy, and lastly adjunctive procedures such as genioplasty, rhinoplasty, uvulopalatopharyngoplasty, or other facial augmentation (**Figure 2**) [2].

2.3 Stock vs. custom prosthesis

There are currently two U.S. Food and Drug Administration (FDA) approved alloplastic temporomandibular total joint systems available for implantation. These include the TMJ Concepts (formerly Techmedica) custom patient-fitted device (TMJ Concepts, Ventura, California) and the Zimmer Biomet (formerly Biomet Lorenz) stock Total TMJ Replacement System (Zimmer Biomet, Jacksonville, Florida). Each of these systems gained approval by the FDA in 1999 and 2005 respectively. The stock Zimmer Biomet prosthesis was granted full FDA approval after completion of a 3-year follow up to an investigational device exemption study which included 442 joints [13]. In several other countries outside of the United States, the Biomet patient-matched, or "custom" Total TMJ Replacement System is available, with which several authors have reported statistically significant success [3, 14, 15]. At the authors' institution (Toronto, Canada), the Zimmer Biomet patient-matched Total TMJ

DOI: http://dx.doi.org/10.5772/intechopen.1004613

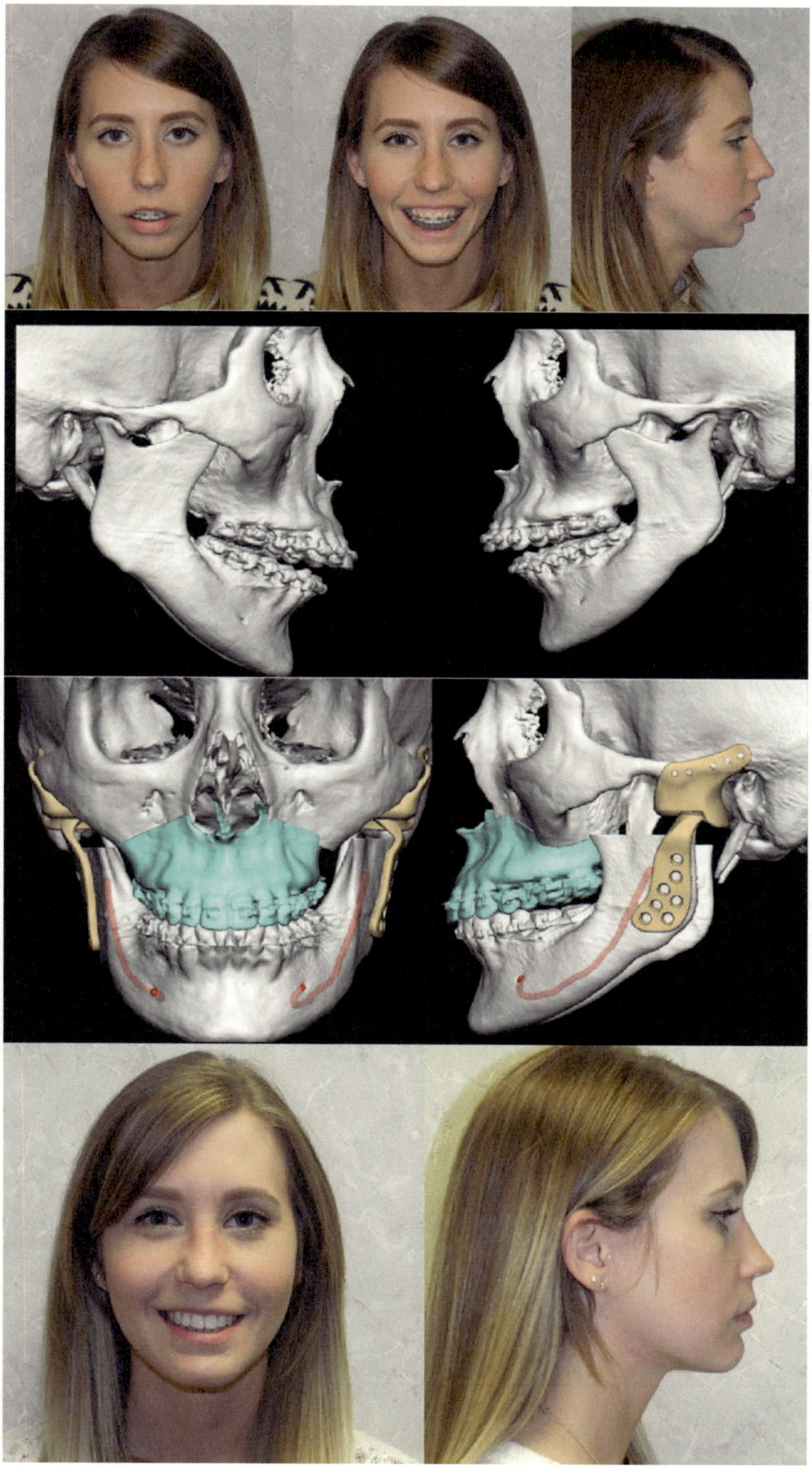

Figure 1.
Patient with severe condylar degeneration secondary to rheumatoid arthritis. CASS was utilized to plan C-TJR-OS. Surgical movements included maxillary advancement and impaction, along with counterclockwise rotation of the maxillofacial complex, flattening of the occlusal plane angle, and concomitant bilateral TMJ TJR.

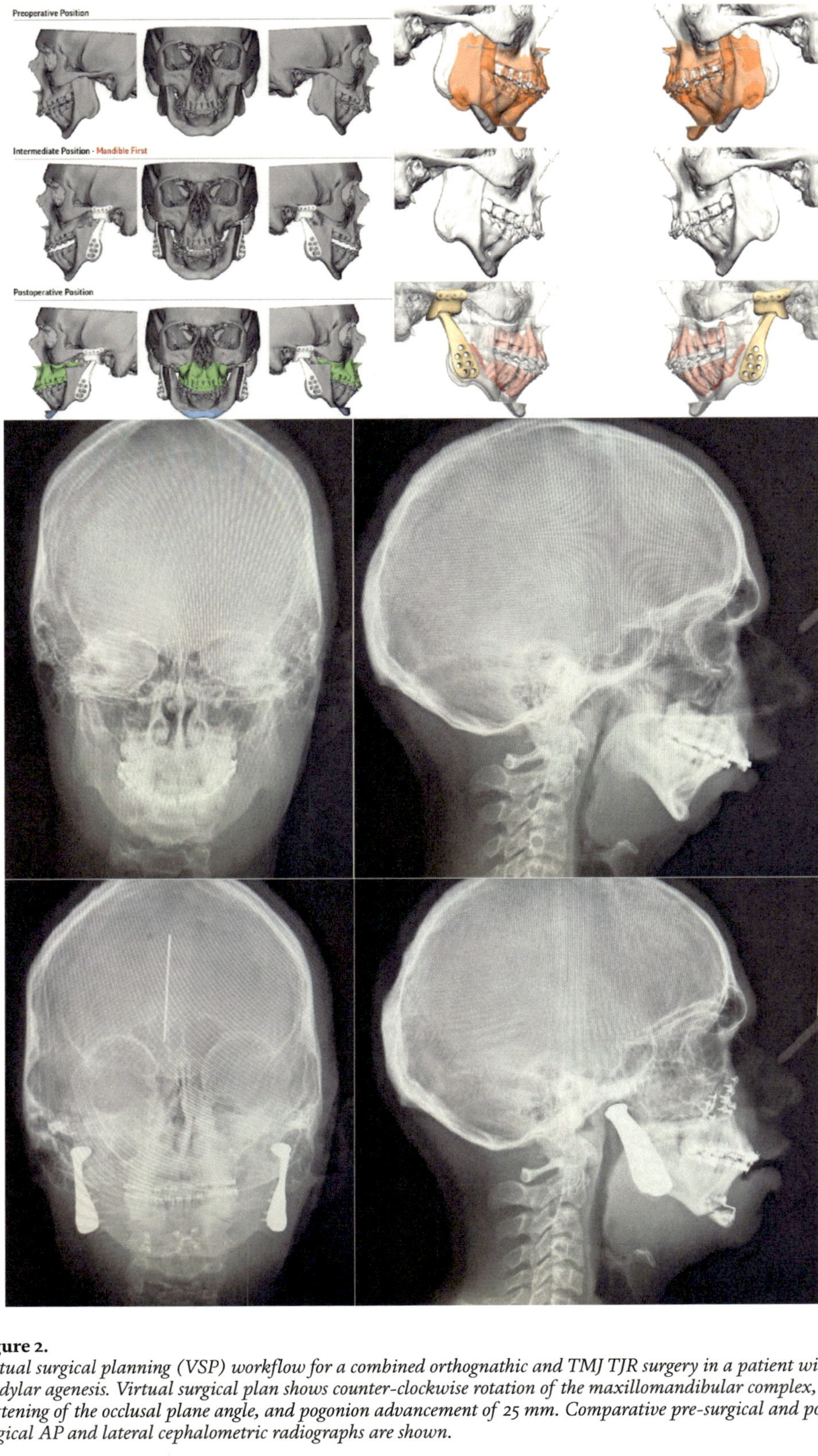

Figure 2.
Virtual surgical planning (VSP) workflow for a combined orthognathic and TMJ TJR surgery in a patient with condylar agenesis. Virtual surgical plan shows counter-clockwise rotation of the maxillomandibular complex, flattening of the occlusal plane angle, and pogonion advancement of 25 mm. Comparative pre-surgical and post-surgical AP and lateral cephalometric radiographs are shown.

Replacement System receives approval on a case-by-case basis after special application to Health Canada.

Deciding between stock versus custom prostheses requires careful consideration of the advantages and disadvantages. The main advantages of stock prostheses are their immediate availability, fit flexibility, and lower cost than their custom counterparts [2]. Provided sufficient bone stock is available for the stabilization and fixation of stock components, these features make stock prostheses particularly useful in cases of irreparable trauma or tumor resection. However, stock prostheses have limited potential for anteroinferior movement of the mandible, therefore surgeon experience is an important factor in managing the variability of fit. Custom prosthetic joints, on the other hand, can address significantly distorted or anatomically unstable situations including excessive antero-inferior movement of the mandibular complex (**Figure 3**) [2]. Computer-assisted surgical simulation of patient-specific implants facilitates fabrication of prostheses which conform intimately to the patient's existing anatomy, ensures optimal implant positioning and the avoidance of vital structures, and concomitant correction of facial contour (**Figures 4–6**) [3]. Unfortunately, these advantages come at a higher cost and a significant fabrication time of 8–12 weeks. Furthermore, there is limited flexibility in the surgical implantation of custom prostheses as surgeons must replicate model surgery exactly. In 2021, Brown et al. found 74% of cases in a study of 241 joints could be adapted to a stock prosthesis [16]. From their research, they concluded that custom TJR devices should be the gold standard in cases requiring a large mandibular advancement with counter-clockwise rotation of the mandibular plane angle, creating a gap of greater than 35 mm between the fossa and the ascending ramus [16]. Furthermore, custom prostheses should also be preferred in cases with severe mandibular dysplasia, syndromic patients, concurrent orthognathic surgery cases, and in the reconstruction of multiply operated joints [16, 17]. Regardless of the differences between stock and custom prostheses, appropriate perioperative planning to ensure intimate and stable adaptation of the alloplastic components is important in the long-term success of these prostheses.

The Zimmer Biomet stock prosthesis fossa (**Figure 7**) is composed of Biomet's ArCom® ultrahigh molecular weight polyethylene (UHMWPE) fossa component,

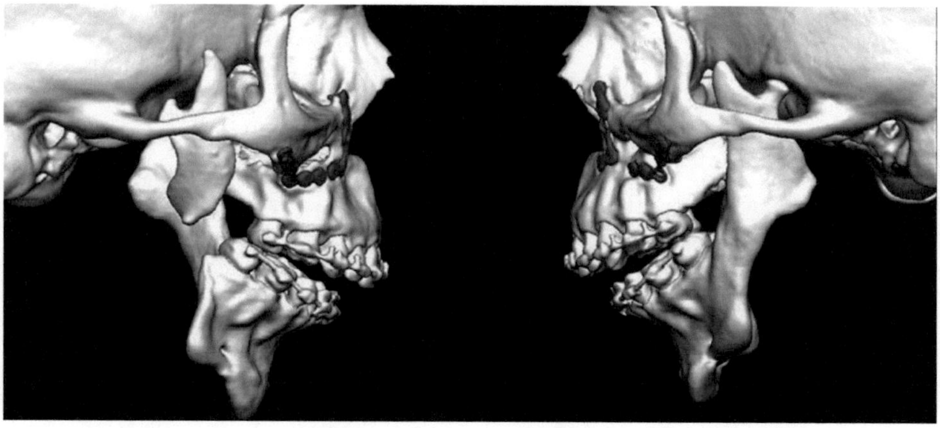

Figure 3.
Preoperative CT images showing a right sided mandibular continuity defect and left sided condylar dislocation into the infratemporal fossa. Maxillary hardware from previous corrective orthognathic surgery is also seen. This aberrant anatomy shown in this image highlights the need for extended patient-matched prostheses for temporomandibular joint reconstruction.

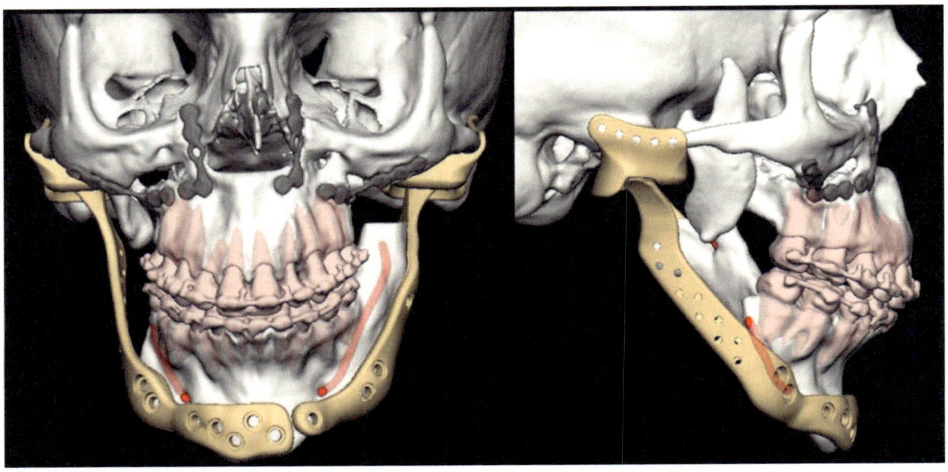

Figure 4.
Computer-assisted surgical simulation (CASS) of the planned osteotomies to re-establish pre-morbid occlusion and placement of extended TJR prostheses. Utilization of virtual surgical planning is necessary for accurate prostheses placement, the avoidance of vital structures, and correction of facial contour.

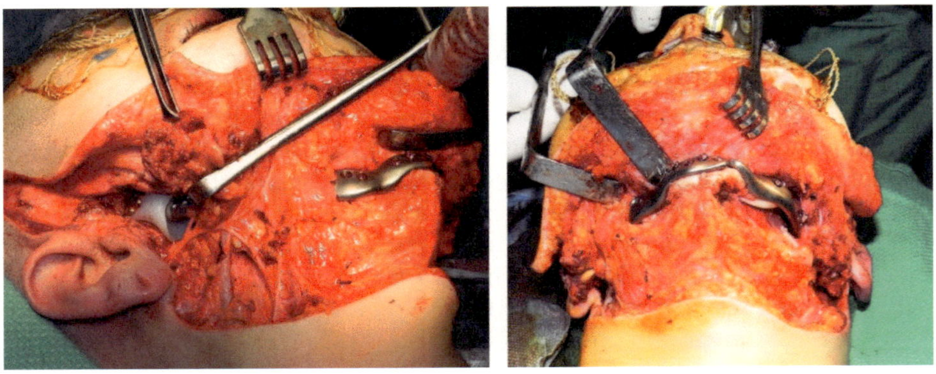

Figure 5.
Intraoperative images of bilateral Zimmer Biomet patient-matched extended temporomandibular joint replacement prostheses.

which is available in three different flange lengths. This UHMWPE is specifically designed to maintain a low coefficient of friction while being characterized by high tensile and shear strength properties, ideal for use in articulating orthopedic alloplastic joints [2]. The UHMWPE is gamma-radiated to increase cross-linking, which decreases wear properties [2]. The small, medium, and large-sized fossa components all share the same thickness, surface area, and geometric configuration of the articulating surface, while varying the anteroposterior length of the zygomatic flange. This variability allows for a differing number of screw fixation sites for the fossa component. Unlike patient-fitted or custom-made devices, which are specifically designed and manufactured for individual anatomy, the stabilization of the stock fossa component relies on appropriate surgical alteration of the articular eminence and lateral aspect of the zygomatic arch to achieve tripod stability. Typically, a diamond rasp is used to perform appropriate eminoplasty. The fossa component is fixated in place using 2.0 mm self-tapping screws.

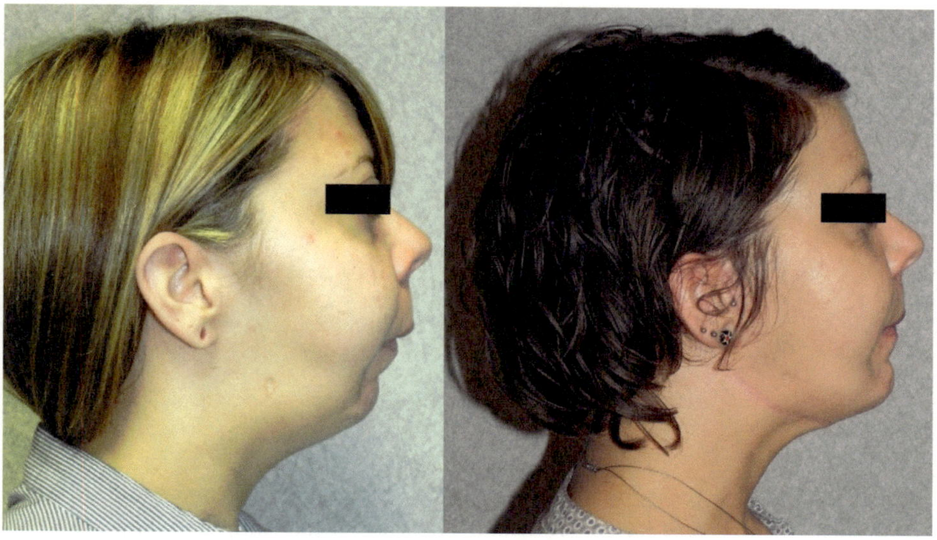

Figure 6.
Comparative pre-surgical and post-surgical images showing improved facial balance and contour.

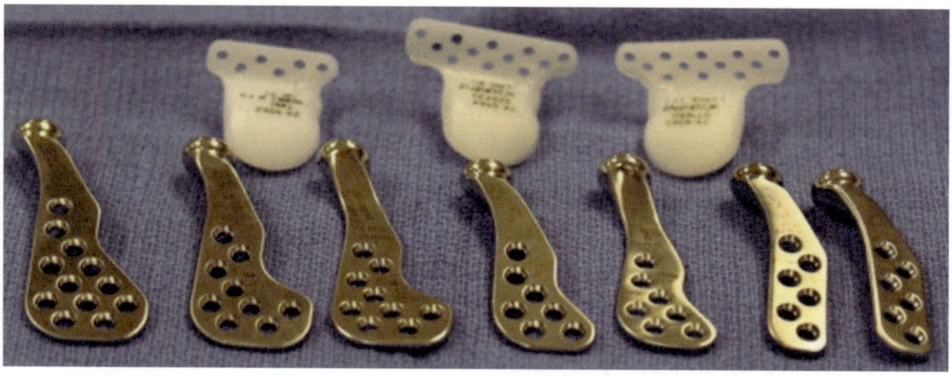

Figure 7.
Zimmer Biomet microfixation stock total TMJ replacement system fossa (top row) and mandibular (bottom row) components.

The Zimmer Biomet stock prosthesis mandibular component (**Figure 7**) is composed of a Co-Cr-Mo alloy (ASTM type F799), which is plasma sprayed on the medial bone-contacting surface with a roughened titanium coating [2, 11]. Much like the stock fossa component, the ramal component is manufactured in three different lengths of 45 mm, 50 mm, and 55 mm. Of note, the 50 mm condylar component is also produced in an "offset" configuration, where the angulation of the condylar head is the opposite of the standard medially angulated head (**Figure 8**). This provides a laterally angulated condylar head for cases where the ramus is medially offset [2]. The ramal footplate also comes in two different designs, either "narrow" or the more commonly used "standard" with a broader ramal plate providing additional screw fixation options. The variability in screw placement is especially important in patients who may have altered anatomy secondary to previous chostochondral grafts or failed alloplastic implants. The mandibular component is fixated in place using 2.7 mm self-tapping bicortical screws.

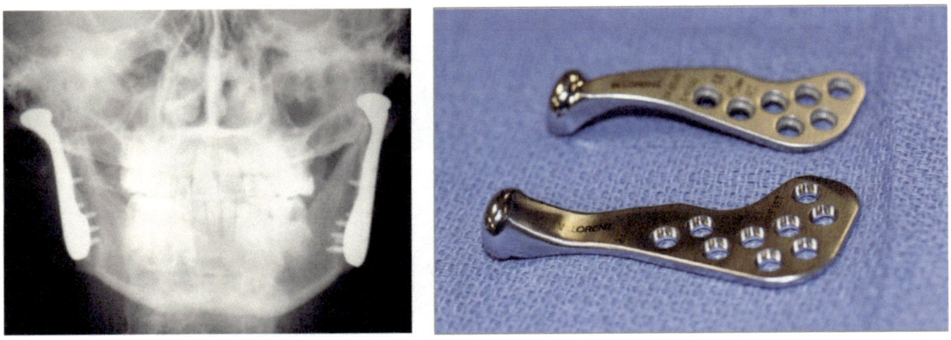

Figure 8.
Zimmer Biomet microfixation stock total TMJ replacement system offset and standard mandibular configurations.

"Patient-fitted" or "custom-made" devices, such as the TMJ Concepts patient-fitted device (TMJ Concepts, Ventura, California), and the Zimmer Biomet (formerly, Biomet Lorenz) patient-matched Total TMJ Replacement Custom System (Zimmer Biomet, Jacksonville, Florida) are designed and manufactured for specific anatomical situations. They often require little to no bony surgical site alteration prior to implantation [2]. Furthermore, with the advent of CAD/CAM technology, extended TJR devices (eTJR) can be developed to replace segmental mandibular defects including skull base defects post-tumor resection or for craniofacial conditions such as hemifacial microsomia or Treacher Collins syndrome [3, 18–21]. Aberrant anatomy, severe occlusal disharmony, and deficient recipient bone stock are surgical challenges that limit the application of stock TMJ TJR in patients needing extended patient-matched prostheses [3].

3. Surgical decision making and techniques

3.1 Pre-surgical planning and preparation

Appropriate pre-operative planning should include a lengthy discussion regarding potential post-operative complications. These include infection, sensory and/or motor nerve dysfunction, foreign body reaction or material hypersensitivity, heterotopic bone formation, dislocation, malocclusion, ongoing post-operative pain, and the possible need for revision [2]. Setting realistic patient expectations regarding surgical goals and outcomes is also an essential element of surgical preparation and informed patient consent. A detailed discussion of expected surgical outcomes, which is outlined later in this chapter, should also be reviewed with patients.

Consideration of comorbid medical conditions and overall patient health should also be included in the surgical planning phase. In patients with end-stage TMJ arthritis related to underlying rheumatologic disease, coordination with rheumatology may be required to arrange perioperative cessation of immunosuppressant medications such as anti-cytokine medication, disease-modifying biologics, or glucocorticoids [2]. Communication with patients' primary care providers is also prudent to ensure chronic conditions such as diabetes or hypertension are stable and well managed prior to surgery.

3.2 Surgical techniques

After appropriate preparation of the surgical field(s), standard retromandibular and preauricular incisions are used to access the mandibular ramus and temporomandibular joint respectively. Regarding the retromandibular incision, a modified Risdon approach is used to expose the entire lateral aspect of the mandibular ramus, the coronoid process, the sigmoid notch, and the neck of the condylar process [4, 9]. Regarding the pre-auricular incision, a modified Al-Kyatt incision is made from the lobe to the top of the helix, with the superior aspect of this incision extending anteriorly and superiorly for about 3–4 cm at a 45° to the zygomatic process of the temporal bone [8]. In the pre-auricular approach, dissection is carried down to the level of the superficial layer of the temporalis fascia above the zygomatic arch and the parotidomasseteric fascia below the zygomatic arch. In close proximity to the tragal ligament, the auriculotemporal nerve and transverse facial artery are sacrificed during the approach [2, 4]. Further dissection is then commenced via incision through the superficial layer of the temporalis fascia superiorly. A fascial flap is then raised anteriorly, typically using periosteal elevators and dissecting scissors, along the zygomatic process of the temporal bone to expose the lateral aspect of the glenoid fossa and the articular tubercle of the temporal bone [2]. Care in preventing tearing or excessive retraction of this tissue should be used to prevent injury to branches of the facial nerve (CNVII) that run through this area. Next, the fossa is entered through the superior aspect of the capsule. Any remnants of the articular disc should be removed at this point, along with condylar resection.

Mandibular ramal osteotomy, and subsequently condylar resection, must be performed to ensure that a minimum of 15–20 mm between the mandibular ramal osteotomy and the height of the articular eminence exists to accommodate the fossa component of the alloplastic joint, depending on the specifications of the device being implanted [2]. At the authors' institution, the mandibular ramus osteotomy including the condylar process, and potentially the coronoid process, is made through the retromandibular incision via reciprocating saw. After the osteotomy is performed, bleeding is controlled and the site is packed with moist gauze. The proximal condyloid process segment is removed through the preauricular incision, and if the coronoid process is being removed, it is removed through the retromandibular incision. To avoid excessive muscular oozing from the temporalis and lateral pterygoid muscular attachments, monopolar electrocautery is used to strip the muscle attachments prior to resection.

Once the condylar process is resected, the residual fossa must be thoroughly debrided before fossa prosthesis fixation. The fossa should be debrided posteriorly to the tympanic plate of the temporal bone, medially towards the medial capsular attachment to the temporal bone, and anteriorly to the anterior-most aspect of the articular eminence of the temporal fossa [2]. Typically, if improper or incomplete fossa preparation has been completed, the alloplastic fossa will not fully seat on the medial aspect, preventing appropriate condylar-fossa relationship upon implantation [2]. If a stock fossa system is used, fossa component stability requires tripod stability which is achieved by flattening the articular eminence with a reciprocating diamond rasp [4]. The fossa should be positioned parallel to the Frankfort horizontal plane, or slightly inferior anteriorly to prevent anterior dislocation. After appropriate fossa preparation, the mandibular ramus may need to be prepared for appropriate passive "flush fit" of the ramal prosthesis [2]. This can be accomplished via diamond reciprocating rasp to remove lateral ramal bony irregularities. Just prior to implantation, the fossa and mandibular prosthetic components should fit passively with appropriate articulating relationship at rest.

Once appropriate occlusion has been set intraorally, with the utmost care being taken not to contaminate the implantation sites, alloplastic component fixation can commence. At this point, the fossa and mandible implants may be seated into position to confirm passive positioning of the implant components. A fossa seating tool or ramus component clamp can be used to assist in orientation and stabilization of the implant components if preferred [2]. Once the components are deemed to be in the appropriate articulating relationship, with the condylar head of the mandibular ramus component centered in fossa in the lateromedial direction and seating against the posterior aspect of the load bearing surface of the fossa, the components are fixated into position using a slow speed guided drill with copious irrigation.

Lastly, after implantation, maxillomandibular fixation is released and the mandible functioned while maintaining the sterility of the implantation sites. When appropriate occlusion and range of motion is noted, training elastics are placed. Imaging confirmation of component alignment, position, and fixation may be undertaken intraoperatively at the discretion of the surgeon, using A-P skull radiographs [2].

3.3 Post-operative management

Post-operative management after alloplastic total temporomandibular joint reconstruction is extremely important and cannot be overlooked. Immediately post-operatively, an auditory canal examination should be undertaken to ensure the integrity of the external auditory canal and tympanic membrane. A Barton-type pressure dressing should be placed, typically to be removed the following morning. Regarding mandibular range of motion, in the immediate and early post-operative periods, limitation of mouth opening may be considered to avoid dislocation, particularly in patients who have undergone coronoidectomies or extensive soft tissue dissection to regain pre-morbid mouth opening or to reposition the mandible [2]. Typically, the risk of dislocation is only a concern for the first week post-operatively. The use of training elastics can reduce the propensity for dislocation [2]. When the risk for dislocation is deemed low, and no immediate component dislocation is noted when the mandible is functioned on the operating table, some clinicians may release guiding elastics as early as 8–12 hours after surgery [2]. Functioning the alloplastic joint as quickly as possible post-operatively will enhance healing and decrease periarticular scar tissue formation which can limit post-operative mouth opening [22]. A significant advantage of alloplastic joint replacement is that patients are typically able to start active physical therapy immediately post-operatively utilizing commercially available jaw exercise devices, such as the Therabite® (Atos Medical, Milwaukee, WI) [1]. Physiotherapy referral to increase and maintain mandibular range of motion may be necessary in the months following alloplastic joint replacement.

4. Outcomes and survivorship

In appropriately selected patients, alloplastic TMJ TJR is a safe, predictable, efficient, and cost-effective treatment option for end-stage temporomandibular joint disease. In 2018, Zhou et al. completed a meta-analysis of the alloplastic TMJ TJR literature that showed both custom and stock devices deliver similar outcomes for decreased pain, improvements in function and diet, and maximum interincisal opening [23]. Like any surgery, reasonable patient expectations are essential for successful joint reconstruction [4]. With careful pre-operative planning and proper placement of alloplastic TMJ TJR devices, patients can be counseled that a post-operative interincisal mouth opening of 30-35 mm is achievable with a total joint prosthesis. Furthermore, a 60–70% reduction in preoperative pain levels and a functional diet 75% of normal are attainable goals with TMJ TJR devices [2]. In an FDA approved Investigational Device Exception (IDE) study published in 2005 on data from 224 cases, Zimmer Biomet noted that patients had significant improvement in pain after 3 years, with pain scores decreasing from 8.5/10 to 2.8/10 [1, 13]. Furthermore, maximum interincisal opening (MIO) improved from 20.1 mm to 29.3 mm at the 3-year mark [1, 13]. Lastly, patient satisfaction scores were high, with 99% of patients stating that they would choose to undergo the surgery again. Wolford et al. published a prospective cohort study in 2015 that reported similarly positive subjective and objective outcomes, as well as improved quality of life in patients with severely degenerated and functionless temporomandibular joints treated with custom TMJR devices at a median of 21 years after surgery [6, 17]. In 2017, Johnson et al. published a systematic review and bias-adjusted meta-analysis of total temporomandibular joint prostheses, including TMJ Concepts prostheses, Biomet prostheses, and Nexus prostheses [24]. The authors concluded that there were no real differences between pain, diet, and MIO scores among the prostheses, although there was more data available for the TMJ Concepts prosthesis [24]. In 2020, a prospective observational study by Granquist et al. noted the Kaplan-Meier survivorship rate of Biomet stock TMJR devices was 96% at 3 years, 94% at 5 years, and 86% at 10 years [25].

5. Complications

As with every surgical procedure, complications may occur that require further management. The most common complications associated with alloplastic temporomandibular joint replacement include, but are not limited to, periprosthetic infection, heterotopic bone formation, dislocation, increasing neuropathic pain, material hypersensitivity, sensory and motor nerve dysfunction, and massive hemorrhage [2]. This section of the chapter will introduce a broad overview of some of the common complications that are seen in TMJ TJR surgery and their management.

In 2011, Mercuri and Psutka published a retrospective survey of 2476 alloplastic temporomandibular joint replacement cases, with 3368 total joints, where 51 periprosthetic joint infections (PJI) occurred, totaling a 1.51% incidence of infection over a mean of 6 months post-operatively [26]. Although the incidence of periprosthetic joint infection is rare, the consequences of this complication can be detrimental. The Musculoskeletal Infection Society (MSIS) workgroup proposed a universal definition for periprosthetic joint infection in 2011 [27]. This definition includes the presence of a sinus tract communicating with the prosthesis, a pathogen isolated by culture from two or more samples obtained from the affected prosthetic joint, and four of the six following criteria:

- elevated serum ESR/serum CRP concentrations
- elevated synovial WBC count

- elevated synovial PMN percentage
- presence of purulence in the affected joint
- isolation of microorganisms in one culture of periprosthetic tissue/fluid
- >5 neutrophils per high-power field in 5 high-power fields observed in a sample for histological analysis of periprosthetic tissue at 400x magnification

Although the detailed management of periprosthetic joint infection (PJI) is outside the scope of this chapter, diagnostic and management algorithms have been outlined based on the existing body of TMJ TJR PJI literature [26, 28–32], as well as the American Academy of Orthopedic Surgeons' (AAOS) Clinical Practice Guidelines for diagnosis of PJI [33]. Practically speaking, periprosthetic joint infections can be dichotomized into either early (within days to <3 weeks) or delayed (>3 weeks) infections, which helps to guide subsequent management decisions. Early PJI are characterized by pain, swelling, redness, and drainage at the surgical site(s), serology showing elevations in ESR and CRP, positive synovial fluid culture with the presence of WBC, and stable components on imaging. The management of early PJI infections typically includes incision and drainage, surgical debridement of the prosthetic components with implant retention, and long-term antibiotics [31]. Late PJI on the other hand, are characterized by pain, swelling, redness, and potentially fistula formation at the surgical site(s). ESR and CRP values may or may not be elevated in these patients. Like early PJI, positive synovial fluid cultures are seen with the presence of WBC, but components typically appear unstable on imaging. The management of late PJI infections typically includes 2-stage prosthetic implant removal, placement of an antibiotic impregnated spacer, and later replacement [31].

Temporomandibular joint heterotopic bone is loosely defined as the abnormal presence of bone in the soft tissue surrounding a total joint reconstruction. Heterotopic bone formation within the joint space decreases interincisal opening and can be a significant cause of pain, joint dysfunction, and eventual progression to ankylosis. Various pharmacologic agents have been used in the management and prophylaxis of heterotopic bone formation, however limited data exists on their effectiveness. Non-steroidal anti-inflammatories such as indomethacin and diphosphonates such as etidronate have been used in the orthopedic literature with varying success [33–35]. Localized low dose (10Gy) ionizing radiation in the initial 4–7 days post-operatively has also been recommended in the management of heterotopic bone formation with success [36]. Concerns have been raised, however, about potential adverse effects on adjacent structures from local radiation. Furthermore, postoperative radiation following autogenous reconstruction with costochondral grafts, gap arthroplasty, or debridement of heterotopic bone has been shown to fail in preventing heterotopic bone formation in 33–50% of cases [37, 38]. Along with surgical excision of heterotopic bone to preserve joint mobility, numerous authors have recommended autogenous fat grafts to be packed around the articulation of the prosthesis to decrease potential recurrences [39, 40]. This obliterates the dead space and prevents the formation of a blood clot. Studies have shown fat grafting around prostheses to be favorable to lack of fat grafting when evaluating heterotopic bone formation, subsequent ankylosis, and maximum interincisal opening [39–43].

As mentioned previously, anterior condylar component dislocation is an immediate and early post-operative concern after alloplastic total temporomandibular joint reconstruction. Typically, dislocation occurs secondary to either concomitant unilateral or bilateral coronoidectomy or due to significant stripping of the mandibular masticatory musculature during the procedure. Immediate post TMJ TJR dislocation is managed with bimanual reduction and placement of light intermaxillary elastics and Barton style pressure bandage for 1 week [2]. Late post TMJ TJR dislocation may require a combination of either general or intravenous sedation along with bimanual reduction. Occasionally, repeat surgical intervention is required to achieve reduction. Posterior dislocation is a rare phenomenon that typically only occurs in patients where a stock TMJ TJR prosthesis without a posterior flange has been placed for concomitant orthognathic surgery [2].

Continued or increasing pain after TMJ TJR can have both extrinsic and intrinsic causes [2]. In the orthopedic literature, post total joint replacement pain can be a significant problem, both clinically and economically, and can vary from between 10 and 50% in the surgical literature [44]. In TMJ TJR, surgeons must be able to systematically rule out and/or manage these intrinsic and extrinsic causes appropriately. Intrinsic causes include, but are not limited to, infection, heterotopic bone formation, dislocation, material sensitivity, aseptic component fracture or failure, osteolysis, neuroma formation, and synovial entrapment syndrome [2]. Extrinsic etiology of post-surgical pain includes chronic centrally mediated pain, neurologic injury, prior misdiagnosis, persistent myofascial pain, complex regional pain syndrome, temporalis tendonitis, Frey's neuralgia, integrin formation, and coronoid impingement [2].

6. Future directions in TMJ reconstruction

The practice of modern oral and maxillofacial surgery, specifically in the treatment of end-stage temporomandibular joint disease, is becoming increasingly impossible without the use of a clinically successful and predictable alloplastic total joint replacement prosthesis. Despite the pitfalls and shortcomings of previous total joint replacement techniques, modern advances in biochemical engineering, material sciences, and our understanding of joint mechanics have made present-day alloplastic TJR devices a safe and effective option for the treatment of end-stage temporomandibular joint disease. In 2016, Onoriobe et al. reported that from 2005 to 2014, there was a 38% increase in TMJ replacement cases performed in the United States. Furthermore, the authors projected that there would be an increased demand (58%) for TMJ TJR devices in the United States by 2030 [45]. As a consequence of increased need, the continued development and improvement of alloplastic temporomandibular joint replacement prostheses is of utmost importance. Undoubtedly, as the demand for TMJ TJR continues to increase, research regarding anatomic and biologic considerations, alloplastic materials, biomedical engineering, design and manufacturing, and the consequences of long-term wear will continue to be necessary [17].

As knowledge in materials science continues to advance, the residual (<1%) nickel in current TJR Co-Cr-Mo alloys is often considered the offending factor in material hypersensitivity. The adverse effects of nickel ions have prompted research and development of high-nitrogen nickel-free austenitic stainless-steel alternatives to currently used Co-Cr-Mo alloys [46–48]. Although Ti6AlV4 alloys have been used with great success in implantable medical devices, there are notable reports of aluminum and/or vanadium hypersensitivity, which have led to the investigation of titanium alloys containing non-toxic elements such as niobium, molybdenum, tantalum, zirconium, and tin [49]. UHMWPE is currently the most used articulating surface material in alloplastic joint replacement devices (including acetabular cups, tibial plateau, and TMJR fossa, etc.) [17]. UHMWPE boasts superior wear performance, durability, and biological inertness [17]. Research into alternate load bearing surfaces include ceramics, which are used in total hip prostheses, and diamond-like coating (DLC), although the appropriateness of these materials has not yet been fully assessed [17].

Other research initiatives focused on advancing TMJ TJR devices for addressing post-implantation complications include the use of human monoclonal antibody component coating to deter biofilm formation and subsequent infection. Another example involves employing acoustic emission detection to monitor micromotion in device components, providing a means to detect potential issues, leading to revision and prevention of premature device failure [50, 51].

7. Conclusion

In conclusion, this chapter was designed to provide a brief overview of the management of severe end-stage temporomandibular joint disease via alloplastic temporomandibular total joint replacement. While conservative management with non-surgical therapies is appropriate first-line treatment for temporomandibular joint disorders, severe anatomic deformity, ankylosis, or loss of function often requires surgical reconstruction to restore form and function. Advances in the field of temporomandibular joint replacement have produced stock and custom patient-fitted alloplastic prosthetic devices that are safe, effective, and reliable. Alloplastic temporomandibular total joint replacement now represents a successful surgical solution with advantages including improved accessibility, reduced operative time, earlier return to mobilization, and lower morbidity risks than past methods. Although research on long-term outcomes is ongoing, a strong body of literature supports the positive outcomes of modern TMJ TJR surgery in patients with late-stage TMJ disease.

Conflict of interest

Dr. David J. Psutka is an occasional consultant and teacher for Zimmer Biomet.
Dr. Ryan J. McCoy has no conflicts of interest to report.

Author details

Ryan J. McCoy[1*] and David J. Psutka[2,3]

1 Fellow in Advanced Temporomandibular Joint and Orthognathic Surgery, University of Toronto, Toronto, Ontario, Canada

2 Mount Sinai Hospital Center for Excellence in TMJ Reconstructive Surgery, Toronto, Ontario, Canada

3 Division of Oral and Maxillofacial Surgery, University of Toronto, Canada

*Address all correspondence to: r.mccoy@mail.utoronto.ca

References

[1] Peterson LJ. In: Miloro M, Ghali GE, Larsen PE, Waite P, Miloro M, Ghali GE, Larsen PE, Waite PD, editors. Peterson's Principles of Oral and Maxillofacial Surgery. 4th ed. Cham: Springer; 2022

[2] Mercuri LG. Temporomandibular Joint Total Joint Replacement—TMJ TJR a Comprehensive Reference for Researchers, Materials Scientists, and Surgeons. 1st ed. Cham: Springer International Publishing; 2016

[3] Boyo A, McKay J, Lebovic G, Psutka DJ. Temporomandibular joint total replacement using the Zimmer Biomet microfixation patient-matched prosthesis results in reduced pain and improved function. Oral Surgery, Oral Medicine, Oral Pathology and Oral Radiology. 2019;**128**(6):572-580

[4] Quinn PD, Granquist EJ, editors. Atlas of Temporomandibular Joint Surgery. 2nd ed. John Wiley Sons: Ames, Iowa; 2015

[5] Mercuri LG. Costochondral graft versus total alloplastic joint for temporomandibular joint reconstruction. Oral and Maxillofacial Surgery Clinics of North America. 2018;**30**(3):335-342

[6] Wolford LM, Mercuri LG, Schneiderman ED, Movahed R, Allen W. Twenty-year follow-up study on a patient-fitted temporomandibular joint prosthesis: The Techmedica/ TMJ concepts device. Journal of Oral and Maxillofacial Surgery. 2015;**73**(5):952-960

[7] Leandro LFL, Ono HY, de Souza Loureiro CC, Marinho K, Garcia Guevara HA. A ten-year experience and follow-up of three hundred patients fitted with the Biomet/ Lorenz microfixation TMJ replacement system. International Journal of Oral and Maxillofacial Surgery. 2013;**42**(8):1007-1013

[8] Quinn PD. Lorenz prosthesis. Oral and Maxillofacial Surgery Clinics of North America. 2000;**12**(1):93-104

[9] Driemel O, Braun S, Müller-Richter UDA, Behr M, Reichert TE, Kunkel M, et al. Historical development of alloplastic temporomandibular joint replacement after 1945 and state of the art. International Journal of Oral and Maxillofacial Surgery. 2009;**38**(9):909-920

[10] Hallab N. Material hypersensitivity. In: Temporomandibular Joint Total Joint Replacement—TMJ TJR. Cham: Springer International Publishing; 2016. pp. 227-249

[11] Mercuri LG. Alloplastic temporomandibular joint reconstruction. Oral Surgery, Oral Medicine, Oral Pathology, Oral Radiology, and Endodontology. 1998;**85**(6):631-637

[12] Mercuri LG, Swift JQ. Considerations for the use of alloplastic temporomandibular joint replacement in the growing patient. Journal of Oral and Maxillofacial Surgery. 2009;**67**(9):1979-1990

[13] Giannakopoulos HE, Sinn DP, Quinn PD. Biomet microfixation temporomandibular joint replacement system: A 3-year follow-up study of patients treated during 1995 to 2005. Journal of Oral and Maxillofacial Surgery. 2012;**70**(4):787-794

[14] Aagaard E, Thygesen T. A prospective, single-centre study

on patient outcomes following temporomandibular joint replacement using a custom-made Biomet TMJ prosthesis. International Journal of Oral and Maxillofacial Surgery. 2014;**43**(10):1229-1235

[15] Fanaras N, Parry NS, Matthews NS. Multidisciplinary approach in the management of absolute trismus with bilateral temporomandibular joint replacements for a patient with juvenile idiopathic arthritis. Journal of Oral and maxillofacial surgery. 2014;**72**(11):2262-2272

[16] Brown ZL, Sarrami S, Perez DE. Will they fit? Determinants of the adaptability of stock TMJ prostheses where custom TMJ prostheses were utilized. International Journal of Oral and Maxillofacial Surgery. 2021;**50**(2):220-226

[17] Mercuri LG. Alloplastic temporomandibular joint replacement—past, present, and future: "Learn from the past, prepare for the future, live in the present." Thomas S. Monson. British Journal of Oral & Maxillofacial Surgery. 2024;**62**(1):91-96

[18] Westermark A, Hedén P, Aagaard E, Cornelius CP. The use of TMJ concepts prostheses to reconstruct patients with major temporomandibular joint and mandibular defects. International Journal of Oral and Maxillofacial Surgery. 2011;**40**(5):487-496

[19] Wolford LM, Bourland TC, Rodrigues D, Perez DE, Limoeiro E. Successful reconstruction of nongrowing Hemifacial Microsomia patients with unilateral temporomandibular joint total joint prosthesis and orthognathic surgery. Journal of Oral and Maxillofacial Surgery. 2012;**70**(12):2835-2853

[20] Cascone P, Vellone V, Ramieri V, Basile E, Tarsitano A, Marchetti C. Reconstruction of the adult Hemifacial Microsomia patient with temporomandibular joint Total joint prosthesis and orthognathic surgery. Case Reports in Surgery. 2018;**2018**:2968983-2968986

[21] Polley JW, Girotto JA, Fahrenkopf MP, Dietze-Fiedler ML, Kelley JP, Taylor JC, et al. Salvage or solution: Alloplastic reconstruction in Hemifacial Microsomia. The Cleft Palate-Craniofacial Journal. 2019;**56**(7):896-901

[22] Turocy R, Salter RB. Continuous passive motion: A biological concept for the healing and regeneration of articular cartilage, ligaments, and tendons. The Journal of Orthopaedic and Sports Physical Therapy. 1993;**18**:639

[23] Zou L, He D, Ellis E. A comparison of clinical follow-up of different total temporomandibular joint replacement prostheses: A systematic review and meta-analysis. Journal of Oral and Maxillofacial Surgery. 2018;**76**(2):294-303

[24] Johnson NR, Roberts MJ, Doi SA, Batstone MD. Total temporomandibular joint replacement prostheses: A systematic review and bias-adjusted meta-analysis. International Journal of Oral and Maxillofacial Surgery. 2017;**46**(1):86-92

[25] Granquist EJ, Bouloux G, Dattilo D, Gonzalez O, Louis PJ, McCain J, et al. Outcomes and survivorship of biomet microfixation total joint replacement system: results from an FDA Postmarket study. Journal of Oral and Maxillofacial Surgery. 2020;**78**(9):1499-1508

[26] Mercuri LG, Psutka D. Perioperative, postoperative, and prophylactic use of antibiotics in alloplastic total temporomandibular joint replacement surgery: A survey and

preliminary guidelines. Journal of Oral & Maxillofacial Surgery. 2011;**69**(8):2106-2111

[27] Parvizi J, Zmistowski B, Berbari EF, Bauer TW, Springer BD, Della Valle CJ, et al. New definition for periprosthetic joint infection: From the workgroup of the musculoskeletal infection society. Clinical Orthopaedics and Related Research. 2011;**469**(11):2992-2994

[28] Mercuri LG. Microbial biofilms: A potential source for alloplastic device failure. Journal of Oral and Maxillofacial Surgery. 2006;**64**(8):1303-1309

[29] Mercuri LG. Temporomandibular joint replacement periprosthetic joint infections: A review of early diagnostic testing options. International Journal of Oral and Maxillofacial Surgery. 2014;**43**(10):1236-1242

[30] Wolford LM, Rodrigues DB, McPhillips A. Management of the infected temporomandibular joint total joint prosthesis. Journal of Oral and Maxillofacial Surgery. 2010;**68**(11):2810-2823

[31] Mercuri LG. Avoiding and managing temporomandibular joint total joint replacement surgical site infections. Journal of Oral and Maxillofacial Surgery. 2012;**70**(10):2280-2289

[32] Parvizi J, Della Valle CJ. AAOS clinical practice guideline: Diagnosis and treatment of periprosthetic joint infections of the hip and knee. Journal of the American Academy of Orthopaedic Surgeons. 2010;**18**(12):771-772

[33] Ritter MA, Gioe TJ. The effect of indomethacin on para-articular ectopic ossification following total hip arthroplasty. Clinical Orthopaedics and Related Research. 1982;**167**(167):113-117

[34] Francis MD, Russell RG, Fleisch H. Diphosphonates inhibit formation of calcium phosphate crystals in vitro and pathological calcification in vivo. Science (American Association for the Advancement of Science). 1969;**165**(3899):1264-1266

[35] Pittenger DE. Heterotopic ossification. Orthopaedic Review. 1991;**20**:33-39

[36] Reid R, Cooke H. Postoperative ionizing radiation in the management of heterotopic bone formation in the temporomandibular joint. Journal of Oral and Maxillofacial Surgery. 1999;**57**(8):900-905

[37] Dolores Durr E, Turlington EG, Foote RL. Radiation treatment of heterotopic bone formation in the temporomandibular joint articulation. International Journal of Radiation Oncology, Biology, Physics. 1993;**27**(4):863-869

[38] Jensen AW, Viozzi CF, Foote RL. Long-term results of radiation prophylaxis for heterotopic ossification in the temporomandibular joint. Journal of Oral and Maxillofacial Surgery. 2010;**68**(5):1100-1105

[39] Wolford LM, Karras SC. Autologous fat transplantation around temporomandibular joint total joint prostheses: Preliminary treatment outcomes. Journal of Oral and Maxillofacial Surgery. 1997;**55**(3):245-251

[40] Mercuri LG, Ali FA, Woolson R. Outcomes of total alloplastic replacement with periarticular autogenous fat grafting for management of reankylosis of the temporomandibular joint. Journal of Oral and Maxillofacial Surgery. 2008;**66**(9):1794-1803

[41] Wolford L, Movahed R, Teschke M, Fimmers R, Havard D, Schneiderman E.

Temporomandibular joint ankylosis can be successfully treated with TMJ concepts patient-fitted total joint prosthesis and autogenous fat grafts. Journal of Oral and Maxillofacial Surgery. 2016;**74**(6):1215-1227

[42] Wolford LM, Morales-Ryan CA, Morales PG, Cassano DS. Autologous fat grafts placed around temporomandibular joint total joint prostheses to prevent heterotopic bone formation. Proceedings—Baylor University Medical Center. 2008;**21**(3):248-254

[43] Wolford LM. Autologous fat grafts placed around temporomandibular joint (TMJ) total joint prostheses to prevent heterotopic bone. In: Autologous Fat Transfer. Berlin, Heidelberg: Springer Berlin Heidelberg; 2009. p. 361-382.

[44] Schnabel A, Pogatzki-Zahn E. Predictors of chronic pain following surgery. What Do We Know? Schmerz (Berlin, Germany). 2010;**24**(5):517

[45] Onoriobe U, Miloro M, Sukotjo C, Mercuri LG, Lotesto A, Eke R. How many temporomandibular joint total joint alloplastic implants will be placed in the United States in 2030? Journal of Oral and Maxillofacial Surgery. 2016;**74**(8):1531-1538

[46] Yang K, Ren Y. Nickel-free austenitic stainless steels for medical applications. Science and Technology of Advanced Materials. 2010;**11**(1):014105-014105

[47] Talha M, Behera CK, Sinha OP. A review on nickel-free nitrogen containing austenitic stainless steels for biomedical applications. Materials Science & Engineering C. 2013;**33**(7):3563-3575

[48] Romanczuk E, Perkowski K, Oksiuta Z. Microstructure, mechanical, and corrosion properties of Ni-free austenitic stainless steel prepared by mechanical alloying and HIPping. Materials. 2019;**12**(20):3416

[49] Haase F, Siemers C, Klinge L, Lu C, Lang P, Lederer S, et al. Aluminum- and Vanadium-free Titanium Alloys for Medical Applications. MATEC Web of Conferences; 2020;**321**:5008

[50] Rogers JV, Hall VL, McOsker CC. Crumbling the castle: Targeting DNABII proteins for collapsing bacterial biofilms as a therapeutic approach to treat disease and combat antimicrobial resistance. Antibiotics (Basel). 2022;**11**(1):104

[51] Ampadi Ramachandran R, Lee C, Zhang L, Supriya MH, Bijukumar D, Pai PS, et al. Total hip replacement monitoring: Numerical models for the acoustic emission technique. Medical & Biological Engineering & Computing. 2022;**60**(5):1497-1510